THE LITTLE BOOK OF THE BIG

ORGASM

MORE TECHNIQUES & GAMES FOR AMAZING ORGASMS THAN YOU COULD POSSIBLY IMAGINE TRYING

SUSAN CRAIN BAKOS

Author of *The Sex Bible*

A QUIVER BOOK

Text © 2008, 2010 by Susan Crain Bakos
Photography © 2008, Quiver

First published in the USA in 2010 by
Quiver, a member of
Quayside Publishing Group
100 Cummings Center
Suite 406-L
Beverly, MA 01915-6101
www.quiverbooks.com

14 13 12 11 10   1 2 3 4 5

ISBN-13: 978-59233-433-9
ISBN-10: 1-59233-433-4

Library of Congress Cataloging-in-
Publication Data available

Cover design: Traffic Design Consultants Ltd.

Printed and bound in Singapore

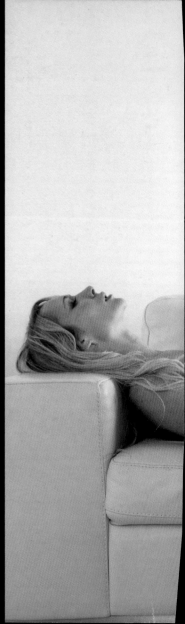

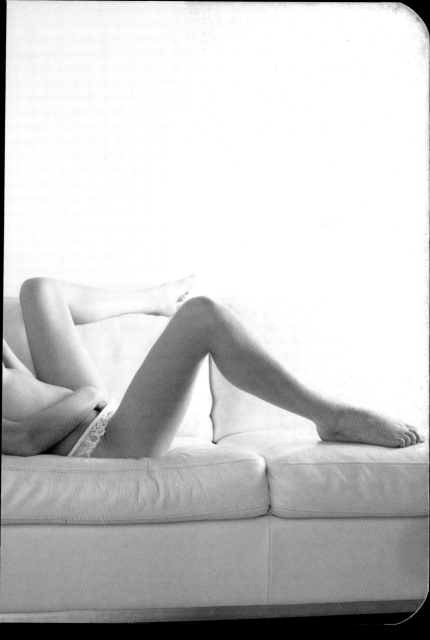

Contents

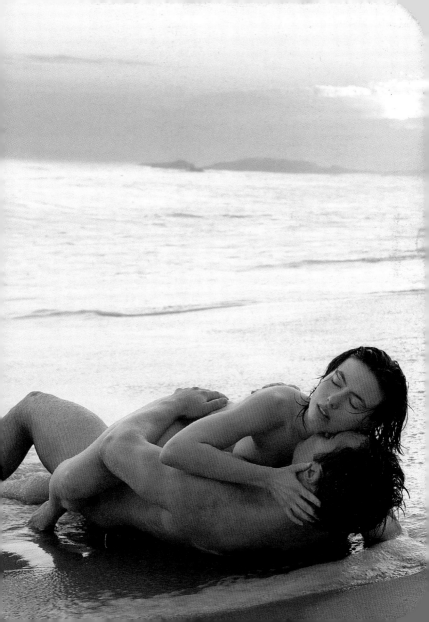

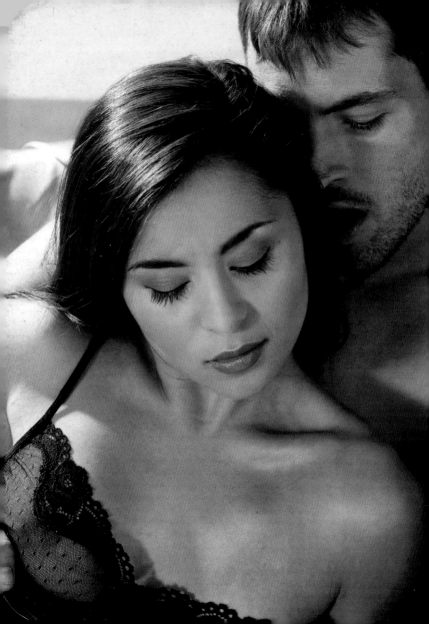

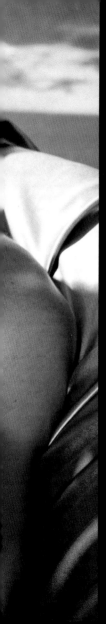

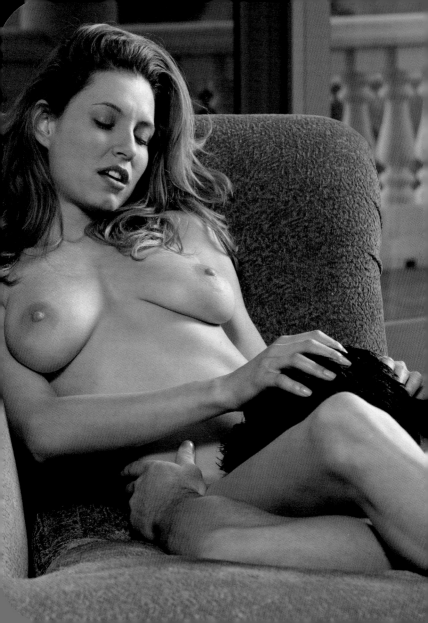

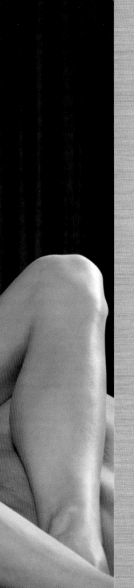

Introduction

For more than twenty years, I have been a sex advisor, writing sex advice columns in magazines from *Penthouse Forum* to *Redbook* as well as books. I have surveyed and interviewed thousands of women and men, and everyone wants to know how to have or give their partner an orgasm. If that's your question, too, then you've come to the right place. This book may be small enough to fit in your handbag, but it's packed with all the advice you'll ever need for getting, receiving, or having as many orgasms as you want. Write to me at sexyprime.typepad.com— and tell me what works for you.

Let's start with some basic anatomy. Now that may sound boring, but the many myths about orgasm may be keeping you from having them.

Truth #1: Female orgasm doesn't usually happen via intercourse alone. Anatomy and physiology are the determining factors here. Most women are not built to get all the stimulation they need to reach orgasm through the friction of intercourse. That friction works great for him. But it will only produce orgasm for her if she is one of approximately 25 percent of women who have what I call an "innie" clitoris. Some belly buttons pop out, some go in. Some clitorises stand out as soon as the woman is excited. Others hide beneath their hoods and the tongue must search for them. All women have an extensive clitoral network of nerve endings reaching into the vaginal walls. Women who reach orgasm during intercourse may have more extensive nerve endings. Here's the bottom line: Intercourse alone will not lead to orgasm in about three-quarters of *all* women.

Orgasms are splendid. They are worth pursuing. Having them makes everyone happier, healthier, and more connected to their own sexuality as well as to their partners. For women, the ability to reach orgasm easily and often is empowering. What's more, good sex and orgasm *creates* intimacy between lovers, something most women really crave.

So if you're one of those 75 percent of women who do not come in intercourse alone, dont be shy about getting what you need—direct clitoral stimulation. Whether it's your own hand, your partner's tongue or finger, or a vibrator you need something other than his penis thrusting in and out of you to reach orgasm.

Truth #2: There's more than one way to have an orgasm. In fact, there are many ways, all of which will be spelled out in this book. But before you jump into the techniques, let me give you a quick tutorial "His and Her Hot Spots." I'll start with yours.

Finding Your Hot Spots

Hot spots are those "magic button" places on your body. You have them. He has them. You know where most of your—and his—hot spots are, but you may not be hitting them (or connecting them with his) in the most effective way possible. If the hot-spot connections are good during foreplay and intercourse, orgasm is more likely to happen and to be more intense.

Explore your hot spots and discover how they react to varying stimuli. You can do this during masturbation, and then take that knowledge into lovemaking, or you can do it together.

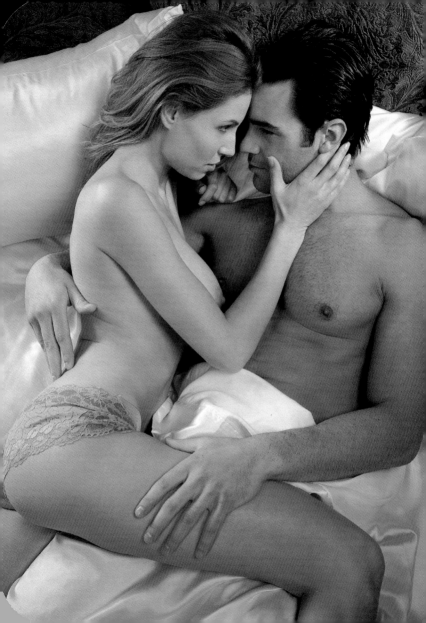

The C-Spot

Nearly all women know that their clitoris (or C spot) is that little pink glans (or head) inside the hood at the top where the labia (vaginal lips) come together. It is sometimes compared to the penis because of its shaftlike shape. For the majority of women, the clitoris and the surrounding tissue is the most sexually sensitive part of the body. The nerve endings of the clitoris actually run deeper into the genitals than you might guess—making this the *hottest* of hot spots.

The G-Spot

The G-spot is that spongy mass of rough tissue located in the front wall of the vagina halfway between the pubic bone and the cervix and below the opening of the urethra. (Because you feel it through the vagina, the G-spot has been erroneously defined as being inside it.) It was named after the German physician Ernst Grafenberg, who "discovered" it in the 1940s, though this spot was familiar territory to the Indian author of the *Kama Sutra* five thousand years earlier.

Can't find it? Place your hand, palm up, at the entrance of your vagina. Insert two fingers and make the "come hither" gesture. Nothing? Try squatting. Some women find it easier to locate their G-spot in that position. Nothing yet?

Use a vibrator, either a special G-spot vibe or an attachment to one you have. That is the simplest and best way to discover the G-spot.

The AFE Zone

Near the G-spot is the AFE zone, a small, sensitive patch of textured, but not rough, skin at the top of the vagina closer to the cervix. Stroking the AFE zone makes almost any woman lubricate immediately. Explore the front wall of your vagina with one finger. When you feel moisture forming beneath your finger, you've hit the AFE zone.

AFE zone stands for anterior fornix erotic zone. A sexologist in Kuala Lumpur, Malaysia, rediscovered this area and named it in 1994. But, again, the *Kama Sutra* got there first.

The U-Spot

We typically don't think of the urethra as a sexy place. But the tiny area of tissue above the opening of the urethra (and right below the clitoris) is a separate pleasure point. Many women stimulate their U spots during masturbation without being aware that they are doing so. Men typically discover it by accident while looking for the clitoris.

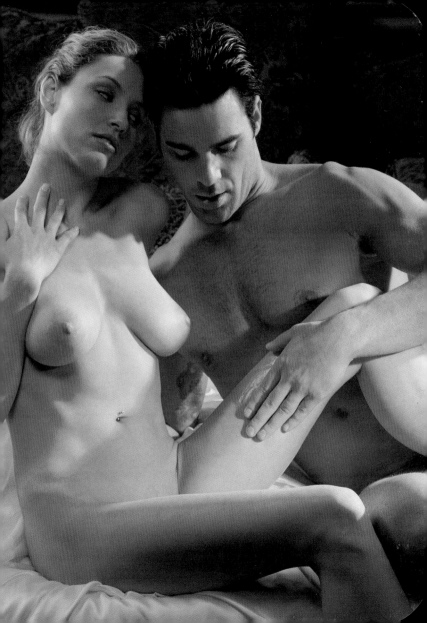

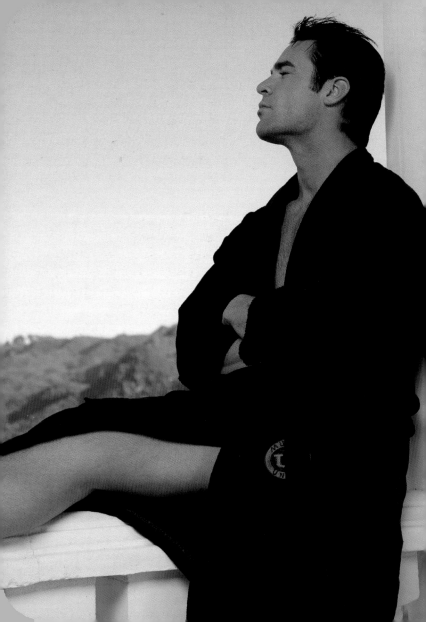

If you've ever thought, "That's not the place, but wait a minute, it feels good," he's hit your U-spot with his finger or tongue. And it's a good place for him to shift his attention between orgasms if your clitoris is too sensitive to the touch for a few moments. Try that after your first orgasm while masturbating.

Individual Hot Spots

Some women have very sensitive breasts, particularly the nipples. Other potential hot spots include the inner thighs, behind the knees, the hollow of the throat, and the back of the neck. After an orgasm, run your fingers along these and other places and see what makes you shiver.

His Hot Spots

Like you, he also has hot spots, those "magic button" places on his body. You know where most of them are. But you may discover a few surprises. Have him masturbate and see how these places respond to different kinds of touch, or use this information as a roadmap to explore his body together.

The H-Spot

The head of the penis is the man's big hot spot, just as the clitoris is yours. Who doesn't know that? Because the head is such a hot deal, the corona, the thick ridge separating the head from the shaft, is often ignored. But it is exquisitely sensitive to touch. Run your finger repeatedly around it. Ask him if that feels good, and chances are he'll say yes. This is why the "silken swirl"— when you swirl your tongue around his corona during fellatio—feels so good. That move, by the way, was a skill practiced by Italian courtesans in centuries past.

The F-Spot

The frenulum is that loose section of skin on the underside of the penis, where the head meets the shaft. In most men it is highly sensitive to touch. Some men reach orgasm more quickly if a woman strums the frenulum during fellatio. If this area feels particularly sensitive to your lover, try that move and see what follows.

The R Area

The raphe is the visible line along the center of the scrotum, an area of the male anatomy too often overlooked during lovemaking. The skin of the scrotum is very sensitive, similar to a woman's labia. Gently run your fingertips along the raphe and see what happens.

The P-Zone

The perineum is an area an inch or so in size between the anus and the base of the scrotum, and it is even more neglected than the raphe. Rich in nerve endings, the perineum is the second-most important hot spot for some men. Use your thumb or finger pad to stimulate it. Start gently and exert a little more pressure if he likes it.

The G-Spot

Yes, men have one, too. It's located inside the body behind the perineum. You can reach his G-spot in two ways: By pressing the perineum with your thumb or finger or by inserting a finger inside his anus and stroking very gently. Many men love G-spot stimulation. Others hate it. You'll know where your lover stands by letting him find it first, or finding it together.

Individual Hot Spots

Like women, men also have individual hot spots, places of great sensitivity that lie outside the genitals. These include the ears, neck, inner thighs, temples, eyelids, nipples, and buttocks. After ejaculation, run your fingers along these places and note any sensitivity. If he shivers, take note.

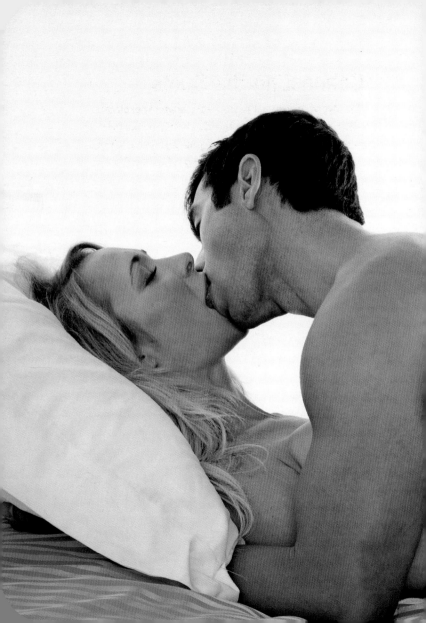

Connecting the Spots

If you've studied—and passed—the anatomy exploration test, either on your own or together with your partner—you're ready for the next step: Exploring the many tips, tricks, and techniques in *The Little Book of the Big Orgasm*.

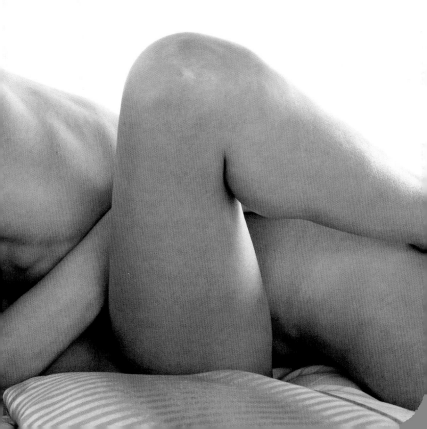

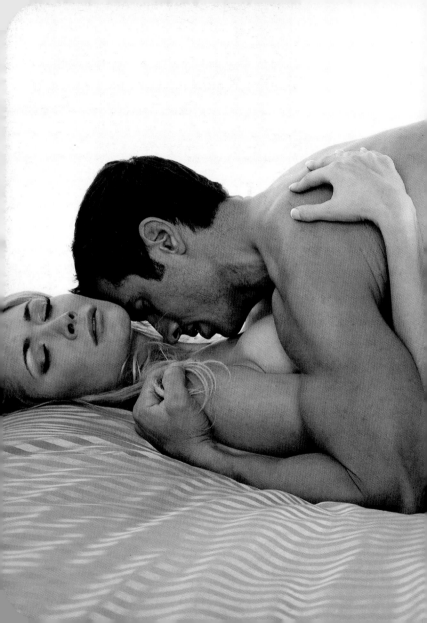

CHAPTER 1

The Orgasm Loop

The Orgasm Loop is a revolutionary mind–body technique for reaching orgasm everytime, any time. The Orgasm Loop taps your arousal potential and teaches you how to use your body to your own best orgasm advantage. Interested in coming more often? Read on.

Getting Started

The first few times you use the Orgasm Loop, you'll have to think about what you're doing. You will need to focus more on achieving arousal and getting your own pleasure than on your partner. (He won't mind. The results will be worth it for both of you—because a man's number-one desire is to "give" his partner an orgasm.) After that, the technique comes naturally—as will your orgasms during intercourse, masturbation, or other kinds of sex play.

What Is the Orgasm Loop?

I invented the Orgasm Loop (or O Loop), a revolutionary mind–body technique, in response to that question I've heard from thousands of women over the past two decades: "How can I have an orgasm during intercourse?" This is the number-one sex concern among women. Everyone who deals with female sexuality for a living hears the question. And we all know the simple answer: Touch yourself during intercourse.

Perhaps a better question is, "Why don't women feel comfortable touching themselves during intercourse?" This is a more complex issue.

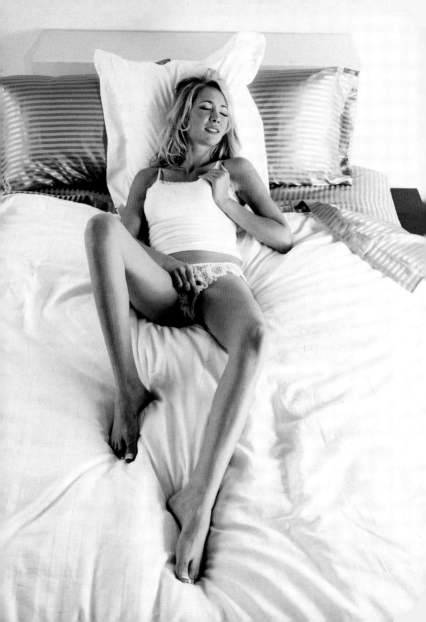

Here are the facts: Women of varying ages and levels of sexual expertise have difficulty reaching orgasm with their partners, and sometimes alone. At least a third of women are reluctant to masturbate, or they do masturbate without touching themselves. (Straddling towels is surprisingly common. Yet no one writes about the problem of chafing.)

While vibrators are increasingly popular sex toys, many women don't know how get the most out of them. And they complain that they either have trouble becoming aroused or sustaining arousal during lovemaking, typically citing distractions like worrying about work or domestic chores when they want to be abandoning themselves to pleasure. That arousal problem compounds their orgasm difficulties.

To develop the Orgasm Loop, I started by researching techniques for removing the mental roadblocks to arousal. Once I discovered the cognitive feedback loop studies conducted by Dr. Eileen Palace at Tulane University, I knew I could simplify the concept, integrate creative visualization, add some adapted sex techniques from Tantra, and take advantage of a woman's natural sexual arousal patterns.

But the Orgasm Loop didn't fully come together until I realized that energy focus—as practiced by experts in martial arts—was the real key to its success.

Here's the bottom line: The Orgasm Loop taps into a woman's arousal potential and teaches her how to use her body to her own best orgasmic advantage. Here's how to do it.

STEP #1:
Visualize Arousal Before You Begin Lovemaking

For women, sex definitely does begin in the mind. Like most women, you may not even know your body is aroused when it is because you won't allow yourself the time to think about sex. Give yourself that time before the foreplay begins. Slip into the bathroom, if necessary. Close your eyes, clear your mind, and visualize arousal as an image, perhaps a color like red or a flower like an orchid or a scene such as the beach at sunset. The secret lies in keeping the image simple, clean, and constant, so that every time you see it in your mind, you think: I am aroused. The more you use the image, the more you condition yourself to be aroused.

And by the way, a mental image of your husband, partner, or lover won't work: You need to tap into arousal as a pure force of its own volition—a force inside you—not a complicated emotion dependent on your feelings at the moment for your partner. Love is complex.

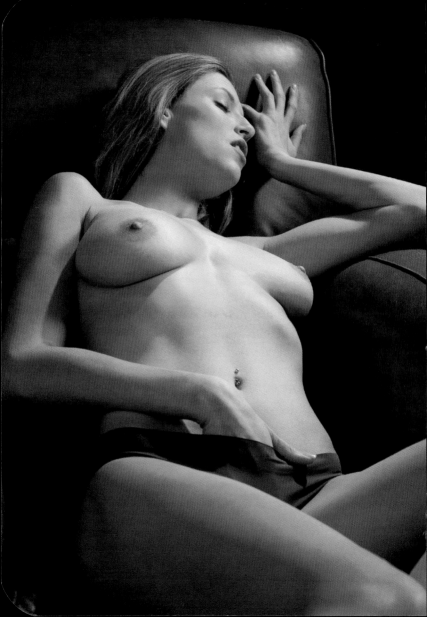

Arousal is simple. You must get inside your own sexual moment before you can be a good partner to him (or her).

An important note: If you are using this step (visualizing arousal) during foreplay with your partner rather than alone, keep your eyes closed as he kisses, caresses, and strokes you, and focus on your mental arousal image. Making love with your eyes open is great—once you are fully aroused. But in this beginning state, you need to focus on your own arousal, not your intense, intimate connection with your partner.

STEP #2:
Focus Energy During Foreplay

Imagine that all the energy in your body is focused in two places: one, a spot slightly below your navel, called the "inner chi" by devotees of Eastern erotic arts because of its proximity to the genitals, and two, the spot at the base of your spine, considered the site of sexual energy by practitioners of Kundalini yoga.

Imagine you are holding energy in those two places until they feel alive with sexual desire. Visualize the energy there. (Just as you can hold your leg or arm out from your body by willing those muscles to perform, you can hold your energy in place.) When you focus on the energy, you feel your body growing hotter and more desirous.

Next, create a circle of fire by breathing deeply
in and out and picturing your breath as fire. Move that
fiery energy in a circular fashion as you draw a deep,
slow breath into your nostrils and mouth. Push the fire
breath down and feel it licking the base of your spine
before you visualize expelling it out of your body through
your genitals.

Do it again. Breathe into your nostrils and mouth
and visualize breathing out through your genitals. See
your breath as a fiery circle that ignites your passion.
Erotic breathing naturally turns up the sexual volume.

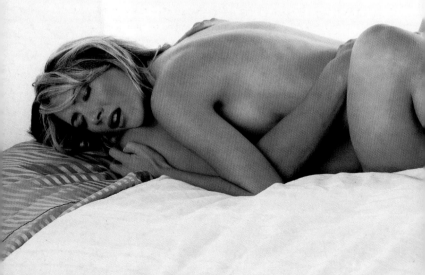

STEP #3:

Move Your Body During Intercourse

Flex your PC muscles in time with your fire breathing. (Not sure what your PC muscles are? See page 34, and Chapter 2, page 61.)

During intercourse, position yourself to make the hot-spot connection (between your clitoris and/or G-spot and the head of his penis), and use your hand for extra stimulation, if necessary. That hot-spot connection triggers orgasm, so use whatever position or leverage you need to get it. Because you have been concentrating so intensely on arousal and sexual energy, you will be more sensitive to erotic touch now than you usually are.

You will reach orgasm quickly.

. . . and Don't Stop

That's right ... if you want another orgasm, don't stop.
Just don't let yourself relax into the postorgasmic state.
Stay in the Orgasm Loop by closing your eyes and going
back to visualizing arousal, followed by energy focusing
and fire breathing. The next orgasm—and the one after
that—will follow.

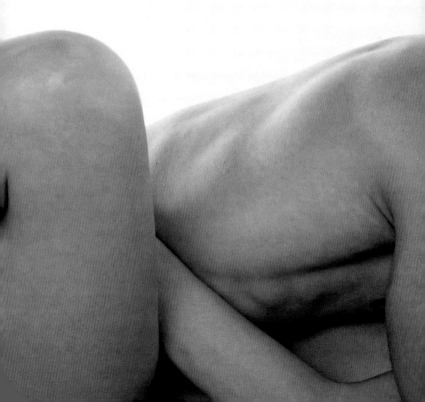

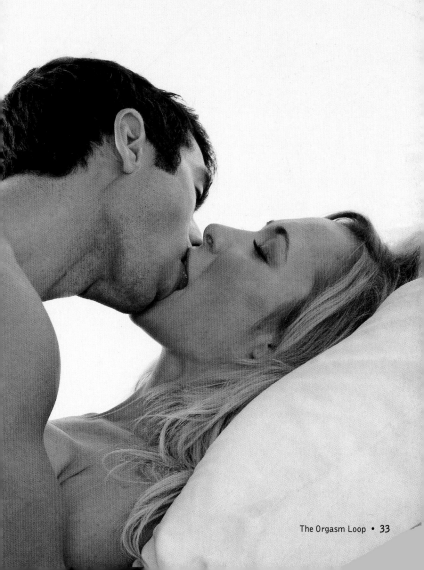

HOW TO LOCATE (AND FLEX!) YOUR PC MUSCLES

The PC muscle, also known as the pubococcygeal muscle, runs from the pubic bone to the tailbone. The PC is located on the pelvic floor and are involved in the contractions experienced during orgasm. Strengthening the PC and gaining voluntary control over the muscle can dramatically improve your sex life.

Identify the PC muscle by stopping and starting the flow of urine. Knowing how to use it to your advantage—can help you orgasm more easily and enjoy stronger orgasms.

Another way to locate your PC muscle, ask your partner to insert a lubricated finger inside your vagina, then squeeze as if you were going to stop the flow of urine. Your lover will feel a tightening around his finger while you squeeze (Exercise the PC muscle by doing Kegel. For more about Kegels exercise, see page 61.)

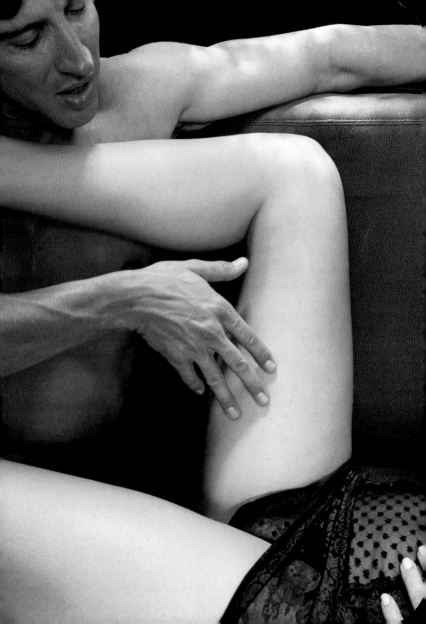

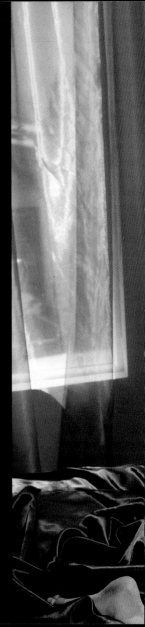

Tap into Two Senses

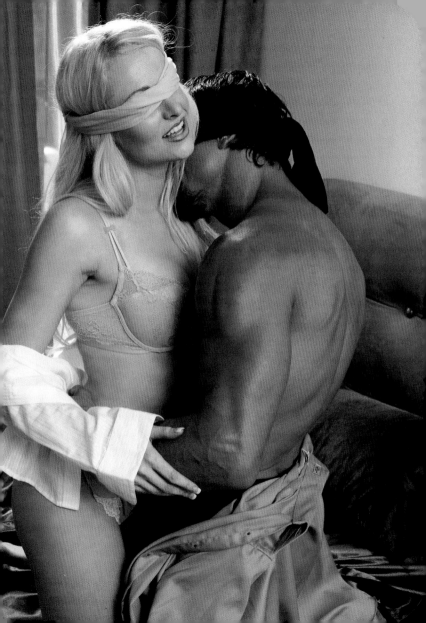

Tap into Two Senses

The Sexy Setup

Text your lover and tell him you need help discovering your special hot spots while you practice your arousal visualization techniques.

Rules & Tools

Select your visual arousal image, such as a red rose, purple orchid, or sunset on a beach. Select a favorite perfume to match your image, or just use a familiar scent. (This isn't the time to try something new. Use a scent that's already known to your lover.) Bring a blindfold or silk ties for gentle bondage if desired.

Playing the Game

Sweet and safe: Before you greet your lover, undress and spray your perfume on any area that you consider a hot spot. Blindfold him and lead him to your bed or a soft rug. Lay down, completely naked, and close your eyes. Practice visualizing your arousal image, but tell him to use only his nose to seek out your hot spots.

Hot and spicy: Pick a favorite beverage or food that smells and tastes good, such as a dab of dessert wine or after-dinner drink or a smear of chocolate or honey. Blindfold your partner and lead him to your bed or soft rug. Prepare your body by dabbing the wine, alcohol, chocolate, or honey on your hot spots, then instruct your lover to lightly tie your hands above your head. Ask him to lick, smell, nuzzle, and kiss his way around your body while you practice your arousal visualization technique. Reward him with tastes of the actual food or sips of your favorite beverage. If he comes up hungry for more reapply and replay as needed!

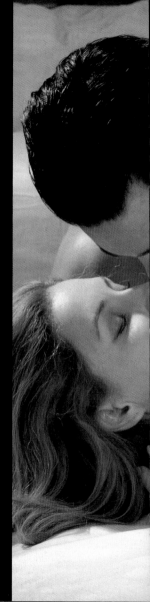

GAME 2

Anatomy Test

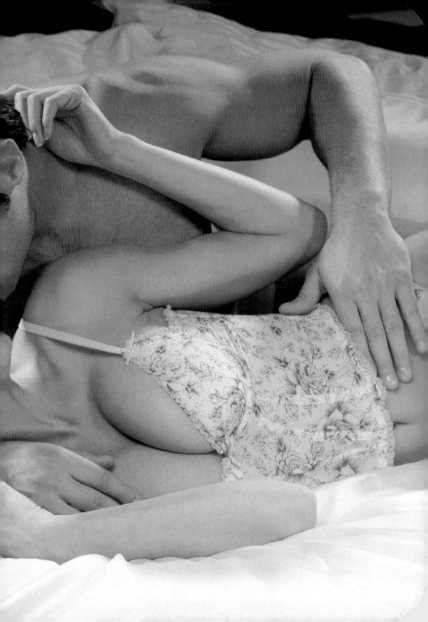

Anatomy Test

The Sexy Setup

It's time for a little hands-on anatomy lesson, and a his-and-her-hot-spot quiz to follow—if you can make it that far!

Rules & Tools

Set up a cozy spot for exploration, such as a soft rug or a freshly made bed. Undress and sit together completely naked. (Alternatively, undress each other slowly with your eyes closed before the next step.) Read the introduction to this book together to learn about all the potential different hot spots. Take notes, make jokes, or come up with sexy names for the various hot spots so you can remember them later on. Bring a blindfold, silk ties for gentle bondage, and edible body paint if desired.

Playing the Game

Sweet and safe: Blindfold your lover and tell him to locate all your various hot spots using only one of the following: his hands, his tongue, his lips, or his fingers. When he's done with his hands, move on one-by-one to his tongue, lips, and fingers. Alternatively, have him blindfold you before he tests his hot-spot knowledge; this allows you to focus completely on your arousal visualization image and enjoy every sensation. Switch places.

Hot and spicy: Before you play the game, use the edible body paint to mark your body with numbers, letters, or other personal symbols, selecting one "marking" per hot spot. Use the order of the markings to indicate which spots are hottest for you, such as #1 for clitoris, #2 for nipples, and so on. Don't forget the less obvious hot spots, such as your lower back, the inside of your wrists, or the base of your throat. Let him blindfold and/or gently restrain you, then call out the numbers or markings to him as he explores your body. For variation, blindfold him and instruct him to visit each mark using his tongue, his finger, or his lips only. Switch places and let him use the paint while you do the exploring!

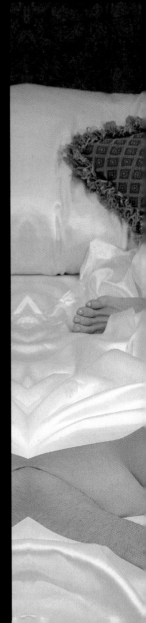

GAME 3

Crisscross Applesauce

(aka Now You've Got the Shivers!)

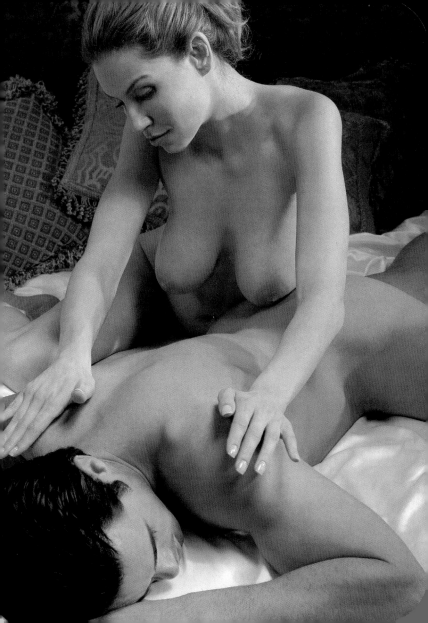

Crisscross Applesauce

(aka Now You've Got the Shivers!)

The Sexy Setup

Remember the children's game Crisscross Applesauce?
Then you know the goal of this game: to bring out the
shivers on your lover's body.

Rules & Tools

All you need is a fingernail, feather, or other small,
gentle scratching device for creating the shivers. Set up
a sensual spot for exploration and keep some paper and
a pen nearby for taking notes. Get naked together in
whatever way you desire or come to the game undressed.

Playing the Game

Sweet and safe: Have your lover lay flat on his stomach.
Straddle his bottom, sitting on his rear end or lower back.
Whisper this rhyme as you make the movements
in parentheses:

Crisscross (draw an X on his back)

applesauce (rub his back lightly in a circular motion
with several fingernails)

Spiders crawling up your back (walk your fingernails
up his back)

Spiders here (tickle gently under his left arm),

spiders there (and under his right)

Spiders even in your hair (lightly tickle his neck,
hairline, and head)

Cool breeze (blow softly at his neckline),

tight squeeze (squeeze his neck or shoulders)

Now you've got the shivers! (run your fingernails up
and down his back or anywhere close by)

Hot and spicy: As you draw the X on his back, gently
sweep your clitoris and labia across his buttocks. Brush
your breasts across his lower back as you walk your
fingers up his back. As you blow softly on his neckline,
run a finger down his spine, around his buttocks, and
back up the crevice; alternatively, whisper "hot air" on
his neckline and press your breasts into his back. For
variation, use the Crisscross Applesauce game on your
lover as he lies on his back and alter the words and
movements to discover where he gets the most goose
bumps sunny side up. Take notes!

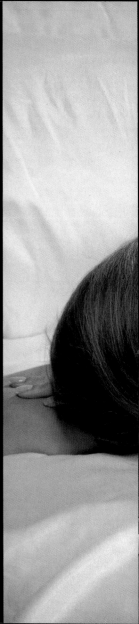

he Art of
eduction

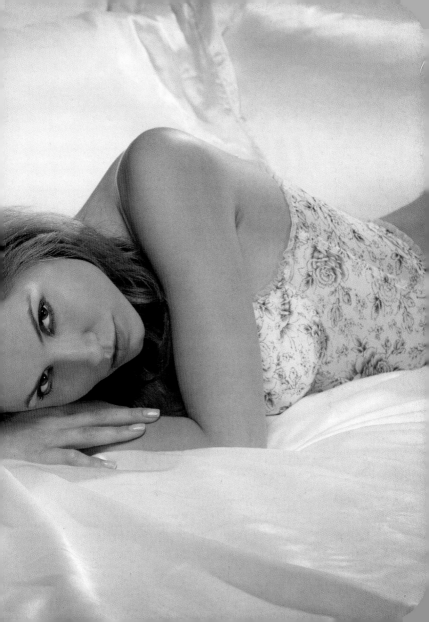

The Art of Seduction

The Sexy Setup

Who says seduction is a lost art? The art of drawn-out flirtation, or sensual interplay between two lovers, can awaken all five of your senses.

Rules & Tools

All you need are a few techniques and someone—your lover or a complete stranger—to practice on. Use your eyes, fingers, and body language to draw your intended victim closer (or create deeper intimacy with a known lover.) This game is best played in an everyday setting; if you set up a sexy scene beforehand, he or she will get wind of what's coming. Instead, make this game a surprise—and the prize is the deep kiss, sizzling foreplay, or extended orgasm that might follow!

Playing the Game

Sweet and safe: Flirting—the foreplay of full-blown seduction—starts with the eyes. Gaze at your lover while he's reading, watching television, or otherwise engaged. Think naughty or seductive thoughts about him until he glances up. As you catch his eye, mischievous thoughts with your eyes...then wink quickly and give a brief smile. (Think subtle) Don't talk unless you have to, and keep your movements and thoughts very simple and sensual. If he glances away, then glances back, play with your hair seductively and let it fall over one eye. Dip your chin slightly but keep your eyes up, then mentally undress him with a penetrating stare. Your eyes will widen slightly at this erotic thought and should, in turn, clue him in to what you're thinking. If he doesn't get the message, move on to the techniques outlined in Hot and Spicy.

Hot and spicy: Use those cliché flirting moves, such as tossing your hair or crossing and uncrossing your legs, to continue sending subliminal messages to your lover. Toussle your hair (as if you just got finished making love) as you gaze into his eyes. Or slowly run your finger from your throat to your cleavage, mentally transmitting your naughty thoughts. Eat finger foods and slowly lick your fingers or lean forward to expose a quick glimpse of your cleavage. If you stand up to go to the bathroom, turn around and wink at him, then swing your hips ever so slightly as you walk away. If you're sitting next to him, lean close and let your breast touch his upper arm. Use these non verbal clues to tease him into submission—or just draw out the flirtation as long as you like!

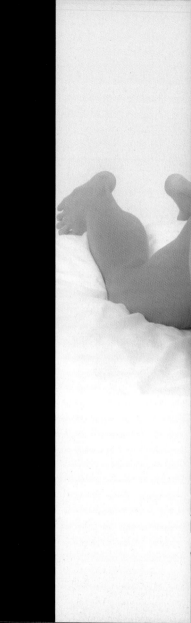

Me Here

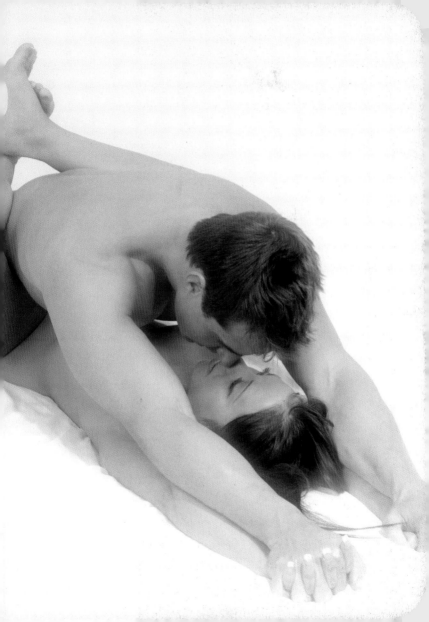

Touch Me Here

The Sexy Setup

This game can be played alone or as a couple, but either way it will help heighten the romance and sensuality in your relationship. Text your lover and tell him you've got a touchy feely game that's sure to pique his interest.

Rules & Tools

This game is about investigating the tools that you and your partner find sexy and stimulating. As you discover what you both like, you'll build a set of props and tools to use over and over in your love play. Wherever you are in your carnal knowledge, start by setting a seductive scene, lighting a few candles, and perhaps opening a bottle of wine or champagne. Keep some beautiful paper and a pen nearby for taking notes, and pull together some sexy fabrics if needed.

Playing the Game

Sweet and safe: Ponder the word "*sensual*" and what it means to both of you. What do you find sexy or stimulating? A cashmere throw? A certain cologne? Ask your partner what he or she finds sensual. Sexy lingerie? You wearing his shirt (and nothing else)? Him brushing or washing your hair? Create a private list for your eyes only. (Over time, the list may grow, change, or evolve.) Take turns practicing (and perfecting) your favorite sensual activities, then set up a weekly or monthly "meeting" to review your list, prioritize your favorites, and experiment with new ideas.

Hot and Spicy: For this version of the game, explore what the word *sensual* means in a tactile way: Play with the fabrics you find the most sensual on bare skin. Pull out your softest cashmere sweater or wrap, silk scarves or gloves, fur accessories, a feather, any other clothing or fabric, then use them to touch and caress each other's bodies. Slowly sweep the silk across his throat, tease his nipples with a caress of velvet, tickle his lower back with a feather, or stroke his penis with a cashmere-covered hand. As you play, don't forget to brush your nipples across his lips, run a finger around his genitals, or lightly kiss his lower back and buttocks. Eventually your travels can lead you to massaging each other with velvet-, fur-, or cashmere-covered hands, stimulating her clitoris with the hint of a silk scarf, or tickling each other's lips, throat, or nipples with a feather. Remember, the better the fabric or object feels on bare skin, the higher the "sizzle" factor (Take mental notes for which fabrics bring out the loudest moans or the most goose bumps)

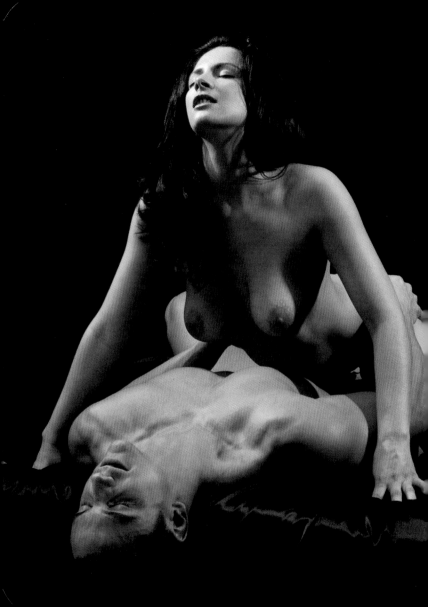

CHAPTER 2

Insatiable Bodies

An *insatiable body* is a healthy, fit body. It gives you more energy for having sex, and the body confidence needed to truly enjoy sex (and let go in orgasms), with an instiable body, you'll have the stamina and endurance to enjoy sex your entire life. What more could body ask for?

The Role of Diet and Exercise in the Lusty Life

Not only does regular, vigorous exercise improve your sex life and increase the likelihood of orgasm, but research has also shown that orgasm is beneficial to your health. Unfortunately, many women are not benefiting from this activity. A large study conducted in 1999, called the National Health and Social Life Survey, disclosed that "sexual problems" affected 43 percent of U.S. women. The top three problems were: lack of desire, difficulty in becoming aroused, and inability to reach orgasm.

Thankfully, such findings often spur additional research, and a later study conducted at the University of Texas in Austin found that women with low sexual arousal who did twenty minutes of aerobic exercise a day, such as fast walking, jogging, or riding a stationary bike, increased their level of arousal and desire.

Regular exercise is just as important in maintaining his lusty life as hers. In fact, as men age past forty, they need to maintain their body to sustain their erection. Excessive drinking and smoking, being overweight, and having high blood pressure can put "weights" on the end of the penis—in other words, bring it down. Viagra and Cialis can help, *but* they leave a telltale flush on your face—and nothing beats a natural high, anyway.

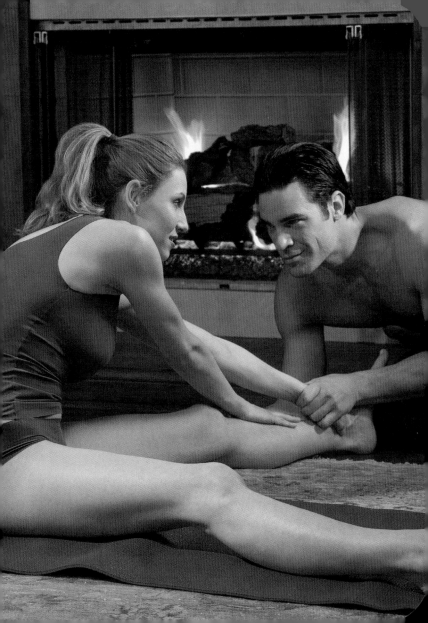

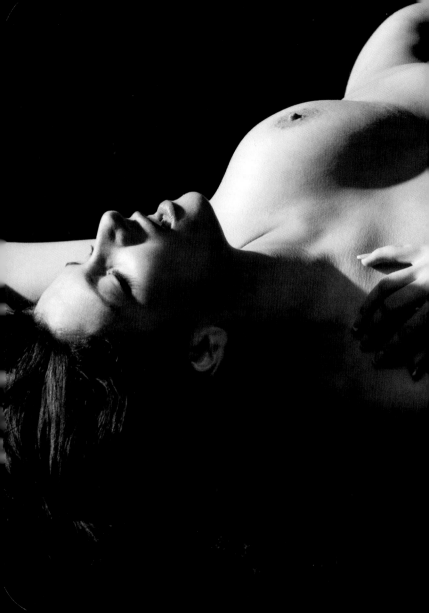

The Indispensable Exercise: Kegels

You cannot have a great sex life with a flaccid pubococcygeus (PC) muscle. It's just not possible. You won't be able to grasp his penis as tightly as you'd like when he's inside you. You won't have the ability to make your orgasm come on faster, longer, and stronger. Without exercising this critical muscle after childbirth, you will never regain sexual tone. (And do you think so many women would need adult diapers if they had a stronger PC?)

Don't skip this section. Do your Kegels. They are critical to your sex life and just not that hard to do. Standing in line, driving, working out, reading a book, watching TV—Kegel time, any time. And yes, he needs that strong PC muscle to sustain intercourse longer and have some control over his ejaculation.

Here's how: The PC muscle is a hammocklike muscle that stretches from the pubic bone to the coccyx (tailbone) in both sexes. It forms the floor of your pelvic cavity. Locate your PC muscle by stopping and starting the flow of urine (but don't do this more than once or twice, as it can lead to other problems. Instead, practice this move when you're not on the toilet.) After you've located the PC muscle, start with a short Kegel sequence, and then add a long Kegel sequence.

Short Kegel Sequence

Contract the muscle twenty times at approximately one squeeze per second. Exhale gently as you tighten only the muscles around your genitals (including the anus) but not the muscles in your buttocks. Don't bear down when you release. Simply let go. Do two sets of twenty twice a day. Gradually build up to two sets of seventy five per day.

Long Kegel Sequence

Hold the muscle contractions for a count of three. Relax between contractions. Work up to holding for ten seconds, then relaxing for ten seconds. Again start with two sets of twenty and build up to two sets of seventy five. Once you are doing three hundred sets a day of the combined short and long sequences, you will be ready to add the push-out.

The Push-Out

After releasing the contraction, push down and out gently, as if you were having a bowel movement with your PC muscle. I said *gently*. It's a slow release of that muscle, with some light pressure exerted while pushing out.

Once you've mastered the push-out, create Kegel sequences that combine long and short repetitions with push-outs. After six weeks of daily sets of three hundred,

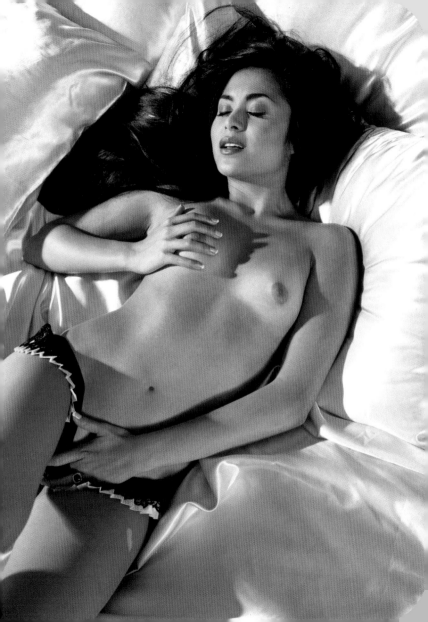

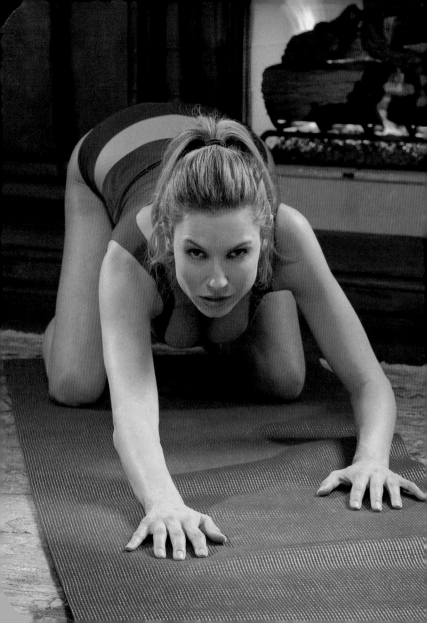

you should have a well-developed PC muscle and can keep it that way by doing a sets of one hundred fifty several times a week."

For Her: The Shag Workout

The Shag Workout is specifically designed to boost your sexual energy and enhance your orgasms as you're toning and trimming. This is a three-stage workout that aims to develop flexibility in the pelvic area and increase sexual confidence, energy, and libido while improving general fitness. Simply put, the Shag is an aerobic workout for pelvic region with some sexual meditation added in. Created by Gymbox in London, the Shag is intense but easy to learn and aims to make you F.A.S.T.E.R., which stands for Flexibility, Agility, Stamina, Tone, Endurance, and Rhythm.

STEP #1: Increase Pelvic Flexibility and Heighten Erotic Awareness

Warm-up: Start with your favorite aerobic activity, for example jazz dancing, cycling, or the treadmill, and do it for 10 minutes. While you're exercising, practice creative visualization. Think hot. Fantasize an erotic encounter or simply concentrate on focusing sexual energy to your genitals.

STEP #2: Intensify and Add Pelvic Techniques

Kick into erotic/aerobic higher gear by adding the following:

The Hot Hips Swivel: After your brief warm-up, stand with your feet about 2 feet apart, your knees slightly bent, and your lower tummy slightly protruding. Put your hands on your waist. Imagine a cone of erotic fire with the tip at your navel spreading throughout your pelvic region. Swivel your hips to the right, front, left, and back in a counterclockwise direction.

Work those hips! Inhale and contract your PC muscles as you move your hips forward. Exhale and release as you move them backward. Move in a dozen smooth, continuous circles. Then reverse direction and do a dozen clockwise swivels.

The Lusty Cat: Get down on all fours. Lean forward with most of your weight on your arms and your butt in the air. Rock only your pelvis for 1 to 3 minutes. Then begin to move slowly across the room like a cat in heat, keeping your belly low but not touching the floor.

As you move forward, lower your head close to the floor and make the motion a cat makes licking up spilled milk, with your head down, then come up slowly. This

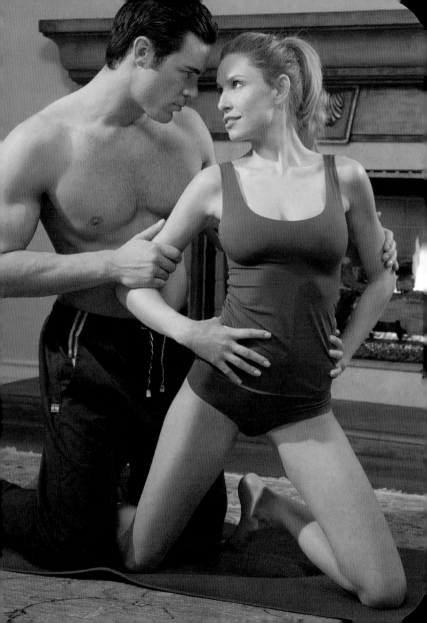

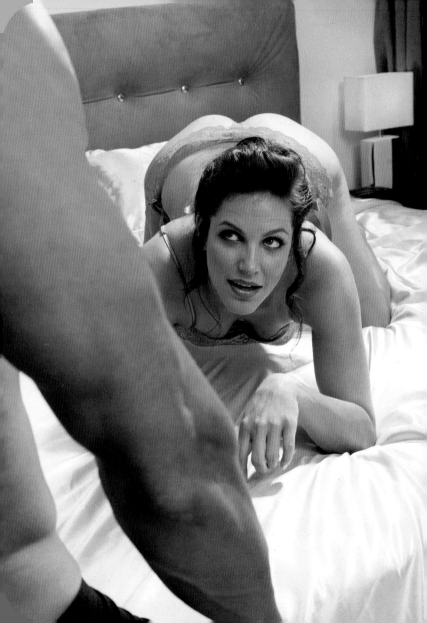

loosens tense muscles in your neck and shoulders and allows the sexual energy to flow up and down your spine. Squeeze your PC muscles and inhale on the downward movement, then release your PC muscle and exhale on the upward movement. Move fast, then slow, keeping your flexes and breathing in time. Do this for 3 to 5 minutes.

STEP #3: Increase Sexual Confidence

This exercise will make you feel sexually alive and more aware of your body, and the feeling will carry on long after the workout. Like other yoga exercises, the Hungry Lioness releases energy in a way that reduces tension. This one specifically combines tension reduction with PC muscle work.

The Hungry Lioness: Get down on all fours. Lean forward with your chest near but not on the floor and your butt in the air. Start a vigorous back-and-forth rocking motion with your pelvis as you keep your chest and back relaxed. The rocking takes place in your pelvis only! Do this for 1 to 3 minutes.

Relax the pelvic muscles and thrust your body forward, with your weight on your arms, like a hungry lioness sensing the presence of her mate. As you lean forward, inhale and gently squeeze your buttocks together. Now push your body back, reapportioning your weight more on your knees than on your arms.

As you exhale, relax your pelvis and buttocks. Repeat the movements for another minute or two.

STEP #4: Increase Your Sexual Energy and Libido

Move back into an aerobic routine like kick-dancing. Regular dancing, even for 10 or 15 minutes two or three times a week, increases your interest in sex while giving you a good cardio workout.

Kick-dancing: Dance to the music and in the style of your choice, but add kicks, as high and as often as you can kick. Jazz dancing is good, too. If you're new to dance, start with modest kicks and build up slowly to avoid injury. Do this for at least 5 minutes, building up to 15 minutes on days you have time for a longer workout.

STEP #5: Relax with Tantra

Use your "winding down" time—and all that released sexual energy—to learn a new sexual technique, such as spreading or "expanding" your orgasm.

Expanding orgasm: Masturbate using a vibrator or your hand. As soon as you become highly aroused, use your other hand to massage the area of your vulva, inner

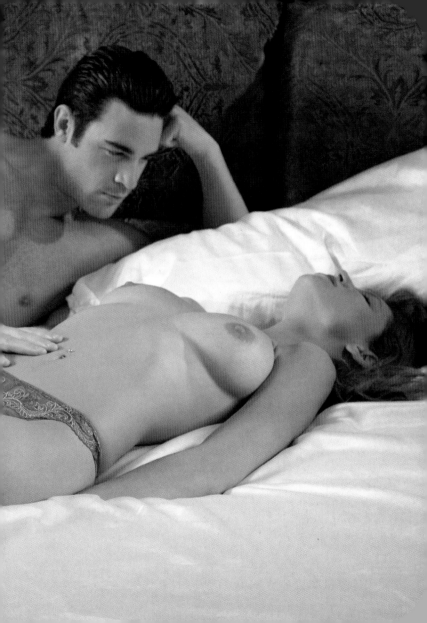

thighs, and groin with light, shallow strokes. Tell yourself that you are spreading arousal throughout your genitals and entire pelvic region. Continuing massaging during your orgasm, imagining that you are spreading the orgasm through your whole body.

After orgasm, continue stimulating your genitals. You will feel the orgasm continue to spread, and you will probably have another or several orgasms, perhaps smaller ones that feel like aftershocks. Some women report actually feeling the orgasm from the top of their heads to the soles of their feet.

STEP #6: Meditate

That's sexual meditation. Close your eyes. Breathe deeply and slowly. As you breathe, focus your mind on the sexual experience you've just had. Now put your man into the picture. Imagine yourself practicing this new technique with him tonight.

For Both of You: Kundalini Yoga

Kundalini is an area of sexual energy within your body. It is often symbolized by a serpent coiled into three and a half circles with its tail in its mouth. Some experts have told me that it sits in your back, in an inverted triangle below your waist with the tip resting above your tailbone. Others have said that the seat of Kundalini is the navel chakra, a place beginning 2 to 3 inches below the belly button and ending above the genitals.

As any true Yogi master would say: Experience it for yourself. Whether you feel it sitting in your back or your belly, focus on unfurling and spreading that energy into your genitals. Your Kundalini and your PC muscle will take you places you didn't think you could go.

Unlike other forms of yoga, Kundalini does not require that you assume defined poses. Start in a simple yoga pose, standing with your feet apart, knees slightly bent, and eyes down.

Freeing the Kundalini Energy: Exhale deeply. Imagine yourself collapsing more deeply into your Kundalini seat with each exhalation. Close your eyes. As you inhale slowly, raise you head, and feel the Kundalini energy rising. Let your hands float at your sides. Now, exhale, letting your head come down again. As you continue breathing, let your body move any way it wants to move. Feel the energy and flow with it.

Do the Freeing the Kundalini Energy exercise side by side or facing one another.

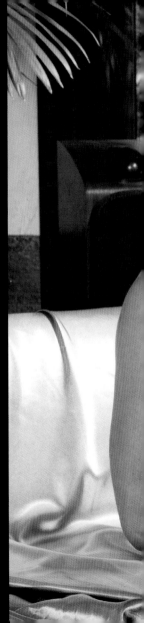

GAME 6

Flex Test

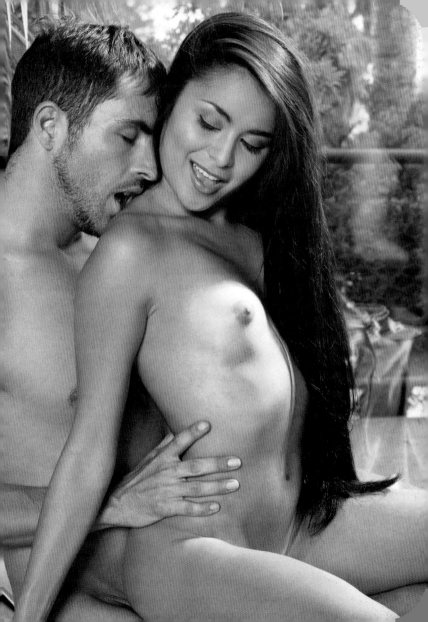

Flex Test

The Sexy Setup

Text or email your lover and tell him you need to work out—but it's your PC muscles that need exercise, and you need *him* as your personal trainer.

Rules & Tools

You can play this game with your own finger, your lover's finger, a vibrator, a set of Kegel exercisers, such as Candida Royalle's little barbell, or your lover's penis. Bring lubrication if needed (make sure you're relaxed and/or lubricated before playing).

Playing the Game

Sweet and safe: Get naked together in whatever way suits your mood—alone or with each other. Be sure you're in a frame of mind (and location) where you can concentrate, as this exercise takes some focus. Ask your partner to help you get excited, but don't go too far—you want to be wet (naturally or with lubrication) but not begging for release. Then settle back in a comfortable place, close your eyes, and practice using your PC muscles while your partner watches—or assists. Start with your partner's finger: Practice pulling his finger into your vagina using your PC muscles, then expel it the same way. Pull in, then push out. When you've mastered that move, try it with the little barbell. In and out, in and out. If this is your first time, don't overwork your muscles—hand the reins over to your partner and let him take over from there! Alternatively, practice on any of the toys, but let him kiss your nipples or finger your clitoris at the same time for a double-barreled sensation.

Hot and spicy: Practice the same moves, but this time use your lover's erect penis or a vibrator. Try quick, rhythmic pulses....then long, slow squeezing. If this move is new to you, try sitting astride your lover and closing your eyes so you can really focus. While it might be hard to tune out all the pleasurable sensations you're feeling, do your best to concentrate on the one move— and ask your lover if he can feel the sensation of your muscles gripping and releasing! Mix up your timing and rhythm depending on what feels good. If he comes close to orgasm, pull away to draw out the sensation and prolong the pleasure.

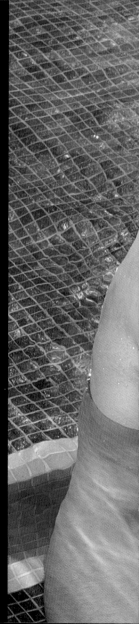

GAME 7

Bring Out
the Big Cats

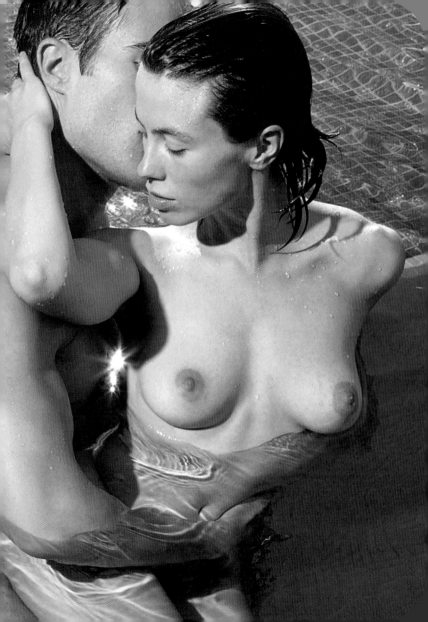

Bring Out the Big Cats

The Sexy Setup

You know you're a tiger in the jungle, and your lover is a lion—better known as King of the Plains. Now use this role-play game to see who rules the bedroom!

Rules & Tools

All you need is yourself, but adding tiger stripes using body paint, wearing tiger-striped lingerie, or messing up your hair and purring softly can heighten the effects! Be sure to ask your lover to play the part of a lion, otherwise known as a big cat who wants to be in charge.

Playing the Game

Sweet and safe: Play like a lusty tigress while your lover watches. Get down on all fours, then lean forward (show off your cleavage!) with your weight on your arms and your butt in the air. Rock your pelvis from side to side, then slowly crawl across the room like a cat in heat. As you crawl closer to your lover, lower your head and slowly lick his toes, ankles, or lower legs. As you travel upward on his body, practice squeezing and releasing your PC muscles and inhaling and exhaling in time. Lick, nibble, and gently bite your way around your lover's body, then reverse roles and let him play the stalking lion. You can be submissive—or battle it out for bedroom domination!

Hot and spicy: Pretend you're a stalking, hungry tigress that's spotted her next meal. Get down on all fours, then lean forward with your breasts near the floor and your butt in the air. Start a vigorous back-and-forth rocking motion with your pelvis and give a gentle growl from your throat. Spot your prey—your lover's penis, his mouth, or his nipples and lean forward, inhale, and gently squeeze your buttocks together. Then push your body back, putting more weight on your knees than on your arms. As you exhale, relax your pelvis and buttocks. Repeat the movements as needed as you move in for the kill!

Playing with Kundalini Fire

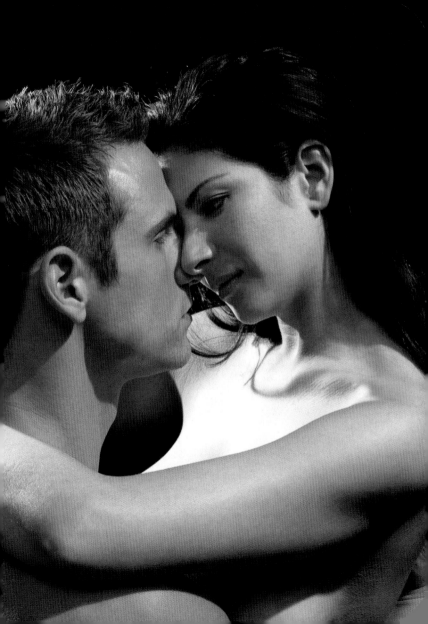

Playing with Kundalini Fire

The Sexy Setup

Text or email your lover and tell her you want to practice some sexual yoga moves together. If she hesitates, remind her that lovers who practice yoga together often come together!

Rules & Tools

Find a large, open space—such as a living room rug or a large blanket in the woods—for your sexual yoga. Wear loose (or little) clothing, and bring along plenty of focus (and a dash of sexual tension!).

Playing the Game

Sweet and safe: *Connecting Energies:* Facing each other with knees bent, make eye contact and breathe together, inhaling and exhaling in time. Open up your arms and hold them around your lover, first without touching. Then hold your partner loosely by the shoulders and breathe together for a few minutes. Feel the sexual energy pulsating through your body and into hers.

Practice this technique while you gently run your fingers up and down her arms, around her lower back, and under her bottom. See how long you can resist kissing each other while you practice breathing, touching, and sharing energy. Reward each other with a long passionate kiss, then try the advanced moves.

Hot and spicy: *Rising Energies:* Face each other at arm's length apart and hold hands. Bounce gently together. Then slowly squat down to the floor. Resting on the balls of your feet, rock gently, supporting each other through your clasped hands. Feel the Kundalini energy uncoiling inside your bodies. Now slowly rise together. As you rise, the Kundalini rises inside each of you. Repeat the squatting and rising, moving rhythmically. After a few times, focus on coordinating your breathing together. Repeat several times, then transfer the energy to your lips for gentle kisses, your hands for lusty caresses, or your genitals for rhythmic pulsing.

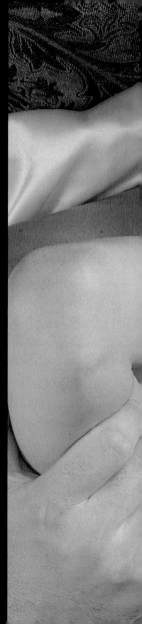

Kissing 101

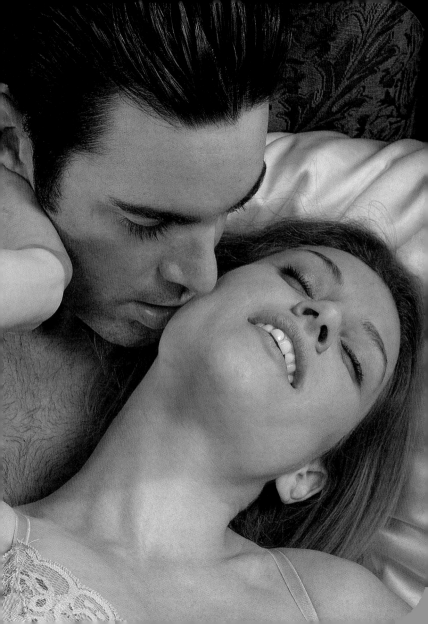

Kissing 101

The Sexy Setup

No matter how long you've been with your current lover or partner, it's never too late to revisit the basics of kissing. Think back to the days when you first met your partner and how you learned what kind of kisses he or she liked, then tell him or her you'd like a refresher course to reignite your intimacy and passion.

Rules & Tools

All you really need for this game is an open mind, a set of healthy lips, and a sense of adventure, but bring along flavored lip glosses, a silk scarf for gentle bondage, or your favorite sex toys for variety.

Playing the Game

Sweet and safe: Pretend that you're meeting your lover for the first time. You've never kissed before, but you know you want each other. Study the shape of his or her lips, noticing if they're thin or full or red or rosy. Outline the shape of her lips with your finger, tracing around her mouth and perhaps stroking her cheek. Ask her what she likes best (or what she likes least) when it comes to liplock. As she describes what she likes, listen, then try to demonstrate like a student following his master. Ask her, "Like this?" Tell her, "Show me." The more you listen—and try to respond in kind—the more she's likely to open up to you, and we all know where that can lead. Ready for more advanced kissing? Lean toward her and use the tip of your tongue to ever so gently tickle her lips, or brush your lips across her lips in a slow and sensual movement. If she's willing, very gently nibble or suck her lower lip, explore the tip of her tongue, or lick her lips.

Hot and spicy: Ready for Kissing 201? Try these techniques. If you'd like her to relax and open her mouth, gently probe with the tip of your tongue. Alternatively, if your partner offers too much tongue, whisper "let's try using just the very tippy top of our tongues" or some other soft and gentle means of redirecting the kissing play. When you're ready, practice (or reinvent) the art of French kissing. Alternatively, have her apply flavored lip gloss so you can guess the flavor—and explore new sensations! Next up: Back her against a wall, hold her hands above her head, and explore her mouth, neck, and cleavage with your lips, tongue, and mouth. And last but not least, come back to the kiss—deep or gentle, light or hard—that makes her melt inside.

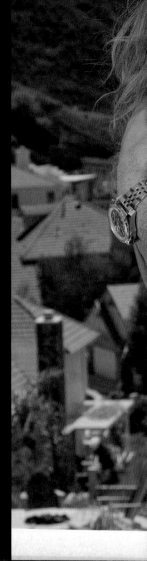

GAME 10

Bump and Grind

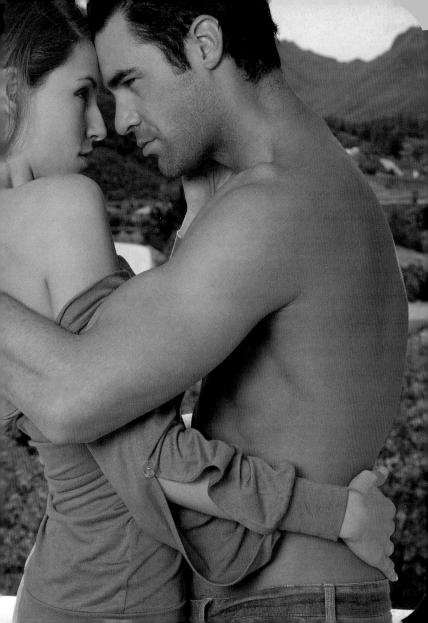

Bump and Grind

The Sexy Setup

Take a trip back in time for this game: Back to the days when making out (not oral sex!) was considered "fast" and "going all the way" was something you *might* save for marriage.

Rules & Tools

All you need for this game is a healthy dose of restraint—and I don't mean bondage! You may want to select your attire depending on how you want the game to go: Lightweight tops and short skirts on her, for example, may make it easier to simulate intercourse fully clothed!

Playing the Game

Sweet and safe: Set the rules from the start: This version of the game has to take place fully clothed. You can kiss, fondle, caress, grope, grab, and stimulate each other in any way you desire, but it all has to take place without removing any clothing—*and* standing up. When you feel the steam rising between the two of you, bump against him on the upstroke and grind into him on the downstroke. Wrap one leg around his waist or use a door or wall for balance—but don't lie down. The goal? To orgasm without actually touching bare skin. Then make a modern game of cleaning up—jump in the shower together or take a long, hot bath.

Hot and spicy: Remember when you were a teenager and you made out on the family room floor while your parents were sleeping upstairs? You kept your clothes on—the better for a quick recovery if the parents came in. And it was really hot. This "outercourse" or "dry humping" game is similar to bump and grind, but you simulate any intercourse position you want, whether it's him on top in bed, her on top on the sofa, or grind from behind on the floor! See if you can stop before you reach orgasm, or don't hold back—let the juices flow! Jump in the shower (and throw those clothes in the laundry!) when the game is over.

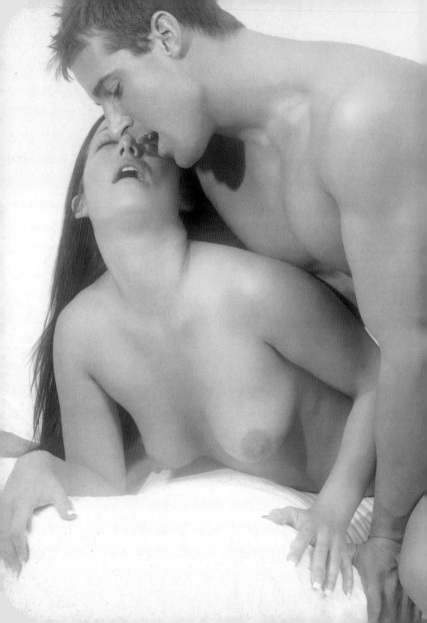

CHAPTER 3

Insatiable Minds

Sex begins in the head—both in the brain and in the mind. Erotic longing, that desire we feel for the another, triggers arousal. And let's be honest: Desire is stronger early in the relationship than it is after familiarity sets in. If you can't sustain it by frequent separations or reignite it by adding "taboo" elements such as discreet cheating or mutually sanctioned liaisons, then you absolutely must heat things up through fantasy, new techniques, and new positions. This chapter will show you how.

Her Insatiable Mind

Women generally claim that they think about sex and fantasize less than men do. Partly, that's a denial issue. Being less obviously connected to their genitals, and thus their arousal, women dismiss or negate sexual thoughts and fantasies. Some women just don't recognize that they're thinking about sex when they are!

Several scientists, including Barry Komisaruk, Carlos Beyer-Flores, and Beverly Whipple, authors of the acclaimed *The Science of Orgasm,* have proven this in the lab. Women who are attached to electrodes measuring arousal, as well as women participating in brain scan research, often show signs of arousal while watching explicit erotic material—even while denying that they're turned on.

In days past, female fantasies had to be obsessively "romantic" to be acceptable. The danger there? The fantasy stopped before the sex really began, and women had even more reason to equate lust with love. But Nancy Friday's 1991 book on women's fantasies, *Woman On Top,* brought the female fantasy out of the closet. The women she interviewed fantasized about S/M, bondage, group sex, rape, and multiple partners. They were just as kinky as their men.

And here's a new trend: Women under forty have more girl-on-girl fantasies, and women under thirty report that as their number one fantasy.

There may be good reason for that: According to a 2006 study in the *Journal of Sex Research*, Australian researchers who studied 19,000 people discovered that 76 percent of women who slept with another woman reached orgasm, compared to only 59 percent of women who slept with men.

What's the bottom line? A rich fantasy life is fertile ground for sex. What follows are some ideas for nurturing her fantasies.

Her Fantastic Fantasies

Women who put sex at or near the top of their "to think" list are women who consistently reach orgasm. Every time you brush aside a sexy thought or an erotic fantasy, you are saying, "I don't have time for my own pleasure." And that's a bad message to keep giving yourself. Instead, indulge your sexy brain. Fantasize, and you will come.

- Read, whether it's erotic, mainstream, or X-rated.

- Watch films with sensual or erotic content.

- Keep a sex journal, recording random randy thoughts, comments on your sex life, and inspirational quotes. You can do this online, but there is something very sensually satisfying about buying a beautiful book and actually putting pen to paper.

- Keep a visual sex journal (or combine this idea with the one above). Collect and paste in photos of sexy men, snippets of erotic art, or your own sketches.

- "Experiment" with fantasies, especially while masturbating. Nothing is taboo, especially when you're alone!

- Dress up for yourself. Try on sexy clothing and prance in front of the mirror. Pretend you're taking part in an erotic photo shoot. Buy new lingerie and model it for yourself.

- Encourage your partner to trigger your fantasies through voice, text, and email messages or handwritten letters and notes.

- Get to know your "favorite friend," or the fantasy that arouses you no matter what.

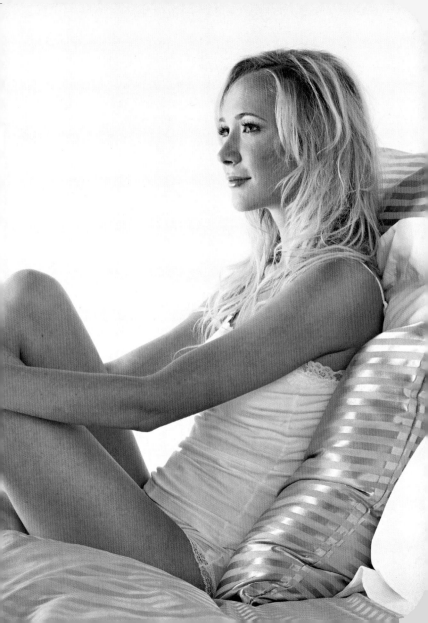

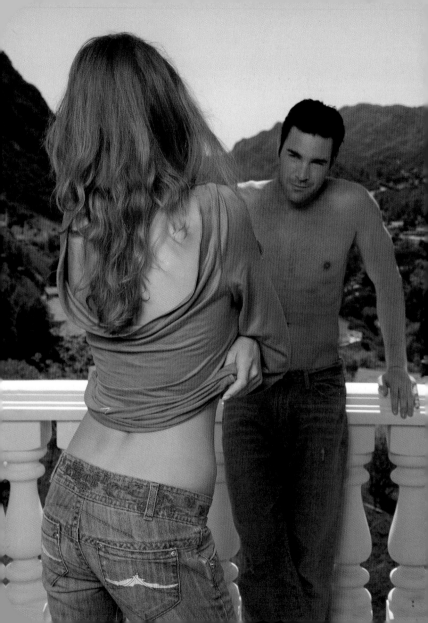

His Insatiable Mind

According to some studies, men think about sex as often as every eleven seconds. Maybe not. But it's often—and the younger the man, the more often it is. Men are much more willing to acknowledge that the fleeting admiration for an attractive person is a sexual thought. Men think: *I'd love to have those legs wrapped around my neck.* Women think: *What a nice tie he's wearing.*

Men do not censor their erotic thoughts. If they are smart, they don't share most of them with their lovers, girlfriends, or wives. They merely delight in them in private.

Women could learn a lot from men.

Fantasy is a nearly universal experience, a mental aphrodisiac with amazing powers. Sometimes it is a conscious process, sometimes not. But if you're not satisfied with your sex life and you aren't using fantasy to create and sustain arousal, you are missing something.

DON'T LET BODY IMAGE
RUIN THE MOMENT

What's one key to good sex? Keeping the mind/brain-to-genital connection snapping like a hot wire in a rainstorm—at least a good part of the time. And here's something that short-circuits the connection: Women will lose their arousal if they catch a glimpse of their less-than-perfect stomach or ass dimples in the mirror while they're having sex. A woman's body-image issues often hold her back sexually, preventing her from relaxing, letting go, and experiencing orgasms.

That doesn't usually happen with men. Men don't think, "Do my thighs look flabby in this position?"

If a man is naked in your bed, then he isn't repulsed by your body. He has a wonderful ability to focus on the parts he likes and let the rest ease into soft focus. And his erection, the sweat on his brow, and the look of lust in his eyes are sure indicators that he has found something he likes. So keep that in mind, and push those body-image demons away—once and for all.

His Fantastic Fantasies

Here are the things men are most likely to fantasize about:

- Something kinky—bondage, S/M, coming on your face, or even worse things he's seen on the Internet, such as a hundred men coming on someone's face.

- Sex with your mother, sister, best friend, or Gwen Stefani.

- Sex with your mother, sister, best friend, or Gwen Stefani—and you.

- Sex acts disconnected from the rest of the body, such as a porn close-up shot of a blow job or anal sex.

- Anal sex with you, like they do it in the porn movies where the guy just "slips it in."

And what does all this mean? Only that he has an active fantasy life. And, yes, he might do some of those things if you'd let him—but probably not sex with your mother unless she is Goldie Hawn. Unless he has nothing but violent fantasies and can't be aroused without them, then he's "normal," whatever that means.

The key to a healthy and robust sex life: to put *both* your fantasies to work.

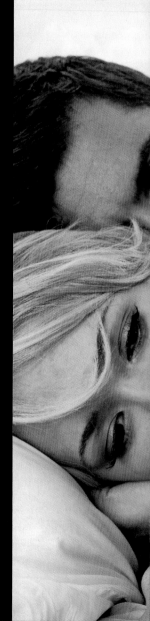

Yourself Off

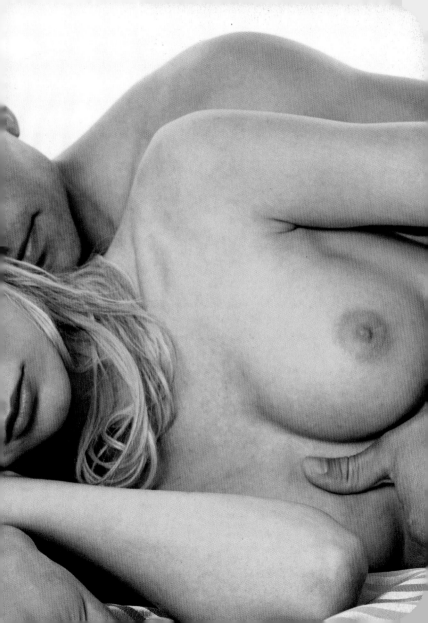

Think Yourself Off

The Sexy Setup

Some women—call them lucky or hypersexed—can have an orgasm just by having their nipples sucked or their inner thighs kissed, and nothing else. An even smaller number of luckier ones can literally "think themselves off," or reach orgasm via fantasy alone. This game lets you try your hand at the ultimate mind-body-fantasy connection!

Rules & Tools

Establish an erotic mood with candles, wine, sexy clothing, or music—whatever turns you on. You can play the sweet and safe version of this game while you're alone, then graduate to the hot and spicy version with your lover. The sweet and safe version can also be used for arousal prior to your lover's arrival—especially if you're having a quickie!

Playing the Game

Sweet and safe: Create a lush, passionate fantasy—and make it graphic. Use your "favorite friend" fantasy if you think that will work best, or come up with something new and daring. Take a dozen deep breaths, then a dozen shallow ones. Use your breath to create and foster your own physical desire. Alternatively, try adding the techniques for The Orgasm Loop from Chapter 1. Flex your PC muscles in time with your panting. As you breath and flex, let your mind relax, having your fantasy help build the sexual desire. If you can't reach orgasm by thought alone, slowly introduce other elements, such as caressing your belly, squeezing your nipples, or palming your "sex mound." Try to hold off from masturbating with your hand or vibrator unless you absolutely have to, and remember that getting even halfway to orgasm is a great start. There's always another day to try, try again!

Hot and spicy: Invite your partner or lover to come along for the ride. You set the ground rules: He or she can watch but not touch; touch in certain instances or places; or jump fully into the game upon your command. Communicate your favorite fantasy, an erotic dream, or a fantastic encounter you've always wanted to have. Take a dozen deep breaths, then a dozen shallow ones. Use your breath as well as visualization, to create physical desire. Flex your PC muscles in time with your panting. Describe what you're imagining in detail to your lover. If it turns you on, have him respond or add his own details. If you can't think yourself off this way, invite your partner to join in at any point to help you orgasm.

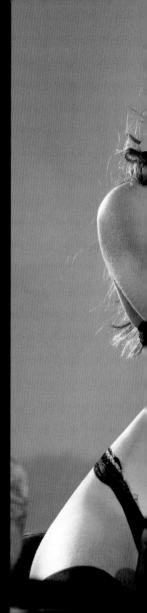

GAME 12

Couple Fantasy Encounters

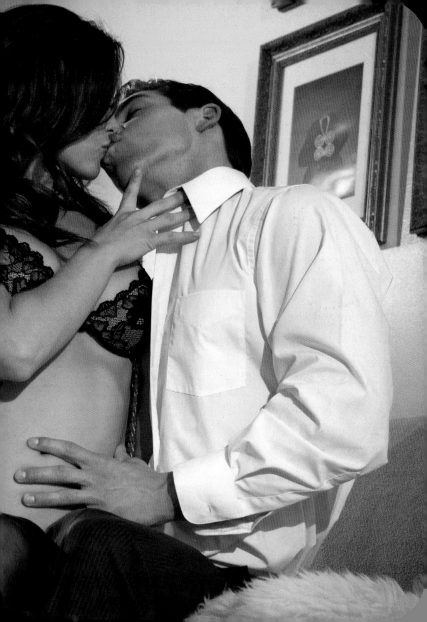

Couple Fantasy Encounters

The Sexy Setup

Tell your lover that the couple that fantasizes together often comes together—and you've got a special game for doing just that. Ask him to start imagining a fantasy the two of you can act out but to be prepared for using more than just his imagination!

Rules & Tools

This game is simple in concept: Create a fantasy and write its script together, then act it out over a one-week time frame. Depending on your fantasy, you may need to assemble or purchase various props. Make a list once you've progressed to the appropriate stage. On the day of the "encounter" be sure to set a private, sensual scene where your couple fantasy can come to life!

Playing the Game

Sweet and safe: On the first night, talk about fantasy scenarios and select one that you both find arousing. (Keep in mind that the fantasy scenario for this game is probably not one of the fantasies that gets you off in private—the key is choosing a fantasy that will arouse *both* of you.) On days two through six, email one another with ideas for the plot, and then take a little time each night before you go to bed to write your script together. If it makes you hot, all the better! (You may want to hold off on having sex during the scripting stage in order to build sexual tension.) Write erotic and descriptive dialogue, such as "The curve of your hips in the candlelight was like a sensuous sliver of the moon in the sky." Don't be afraid to go over the top. Assemble props—masks, costumes, sex toys—ahead of time, or think about playing with edible body paints, food, or other edible props. On the last day, act out your script together as if you were presenting an erotic play—and be prepared for mind-blowing orgasms!

Hot and spicy: There are a variety of ways to spice up this game. Imagine you're creating a magazine article about your fantasy encounter and take photos along the way; envision a storyboard of your fantasy with notes, the script, photos, and props as your building blocks. Alternatively, try filming your actions during the week, culminating with filming your erotic fantasy as you act it out. Ready for even more action? Invite an audience to watch (but not participate). If you're *really* ready to step it up, create and act out a fantasy that includes another woman, another man, or even another couple.

The Queen of Orgasm

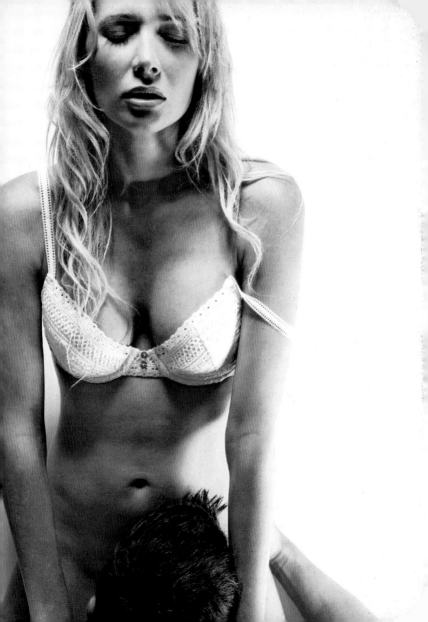

The Queen of Orgasm

The Sexy Setup

Many women fantasize about being dominant, in part because usually it's the male who takes the lead. Here's a game with many different flavors and variations that allows the woman to command the troops!

Rules & Tools

There's only one rule in this game: what *you* say goes. The tools will vary depending on your fantasy: If you're the queen and he's your prince, then pull out an old bridesmaid's dress and act the part. If you're the mistress and he's the sex slave, then pull out those black boots, don a leather jacket, and borrow a riding crop for gentle sex play.

Playing the Game

Sweet and safe: Tell your lover the theme for your domination game, then dress (or undress!) appropriately. You're the boss, and his job is to service you—in whatever way turns you on (and gets you off!) the most. Want him to get on his knees and eat you out? Tell him. Wishing he'd lather your whole body in lotion and massage you to orgasm? Say the word. Want him to watch you masturbate while he films it? Issue your orders!

Hot and spicy: Here's where you can step it up, either by introducing props or letting out your dominant, dirty, or naughty side. When you're wearing boots and leather, use the riding crop for a few gentle taps on his naked behind. If you really like the idea of a sex slave, keep him naked for several hours on a Sunday afternoon—and at your beck and call, whether it's for sex, food, or laundry! Alternatively, have your way with *him*—try tying his hands to the bedposts, then ride him like a cowgirl. Don't let him loose until he's come three times, even if he begs for release. Or tie his hands up and tease him, whether that means stimulating him or yourself (or both)! Whatever gets you (or him) off, make it happen—but remember you're the boss.

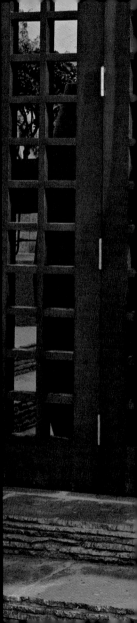

GAME 14

Handyman Cum Calling

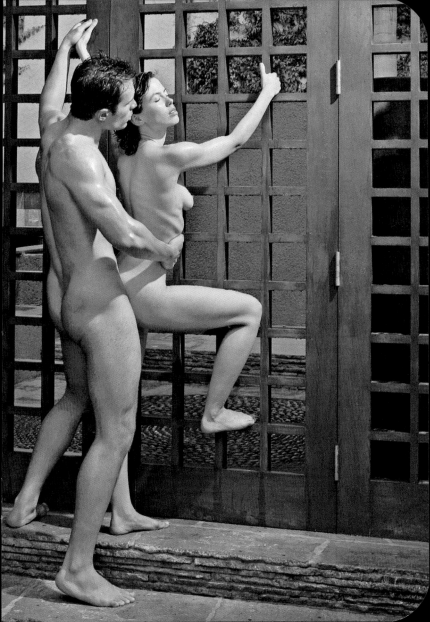

Handyman Cum Calling

The Sexy Setup

This is every stay-at-home mom's fantasy: the hot and randy handyman who's handy in more ways than one! Tell your lover you've got a secret game for her, but you're not going to tell her what it is until the game begins. She doesn't need to do anything special—except be home alone when you come knocking!

Rules & Tools

Dress the part—put on a pair of dirty jeans, work boots, and a big sweatshirt or heavy jacket. Borrow a tool belt and load it up with sex toys, lubricant, or silk ties, but keep it under your jacket or in a bucket or shopping bag so she doesn't see it at first.

Playing the Game

Sweet and safe: Ring the doorbell. When she answers, tell her you're the handyman whose come to help around the house. Ask her what needs fixing. Are her drawers squeaky? Do the bedsprings need attention? Depending on her answer, lead her to the room where you can best play the game, then tell her you're handy in more ways than one. Ask her where your hands are most needed: To undress her slowly? To caress her breasts and nipples? To stimulate her clitoris? Then get to *work*!

Hot and spicy: Ring the doorbell, introduce yourself, and take charge. Lead her from room to room, slowly building the seduction and asking her what she needs fixed. Offer to change the lightbulb, but brush up against her suggestively, kiss her ankles as you pretend to look under the couch, or grab her from behind as she moves from room to room. Once you've settled on a room, take off your coat and show her your tools, then tell her you're especially handy with tools that penetrate, applying lubricant where it's most needed, and screwing things in. Demonstrate just how handy you are until she's hot and wet, then strip down and nail her on the floor. Ready to take it up a notch? Surprise your lover by wearing a tool belt—and nothing else. Make yourself hard before you walk in the room and she's sure to melt at the sight of her favorite tool!

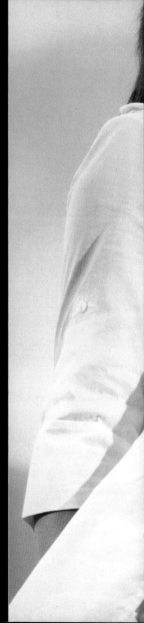

GAME 15

Back to School

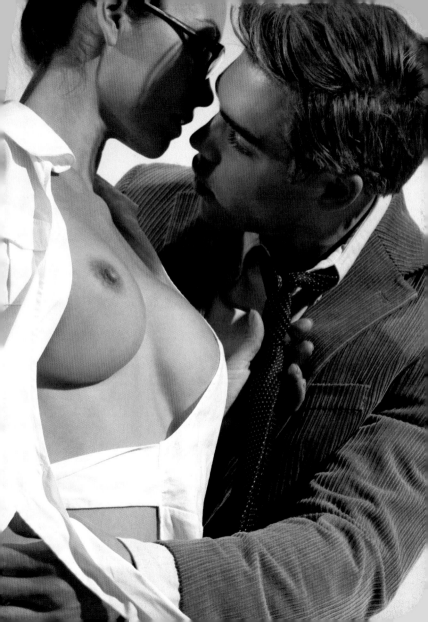

Back to School

The Sexy Setup

Ask your lover if he's ready to return to the schoolhouse, but this time his courses will include some hot and naughty fantasy play! Then get ready to dress up like a schoolgirl or the hot and sexy teacher who he's always fantasized about.

Rules & Tools

To d the part of a schoolgirl, short blue skirt, white blouse, and white knee-highs. If you're feeling really daring, skip the underwear. To play the part of a teacher, try a low-cut white blouse, thigh-high white garters, a skirt, and high heels! Set up the scene beforehand—have a ruler, pencils, notebooks, and a desk ready for your game, and stash lubricant, sex toys, and silk ties in the drawers.

Playing the Game

Sweet and safe (schoolgirl): Invite your lover into the schoolhouse and lead him to his seat, perhaps flashing a glimpse of your upper thigh or bare bottom. Talk him through an overview of your course notes, all the while flouncing your skirt, bending over suggestively, or playing with your hair. Ready to tease him further? Sit on his lap and play with his hair, then put his hand on your thigh and tell him today's lesson is anatomy. To step it up a notch, grab his package, kiss and then pull away, or play with yourself while he watches—then tell him you've been naughty and you need a good spanking!

Hot and spicy (teacher): Pick a lesson for the day—anatomy, biology, even sexual response—and talk about the course as you walk around the room, all the while flashing your leg, leaning over his desk to show your cleavage, or slapping the ruler gently on your hand. As you quiz him on his knowledge, slowly remove your skirt or blouse, all the while staring directly into his eyes. Reward him with a kiss or a touch of your breast if he answers a question correctly, but then move away so the teasing tension continues to build. Continue removing your clothing, then kiss the back of his neck as you stroke his chest from behind, or order him to kiss your breasts, fondle your bottom, stroke your thighs, or even lick your clitoris—but always pull away at some point to continue teasing. Ready for the final exam? Position yourself on the desk and invite him over! Alternatively, surprise him by reversing roles: Get into a gentle struggle (but let him win). Have him tie you to the chair or desk, then either tease you into submission or take you while you fight back.

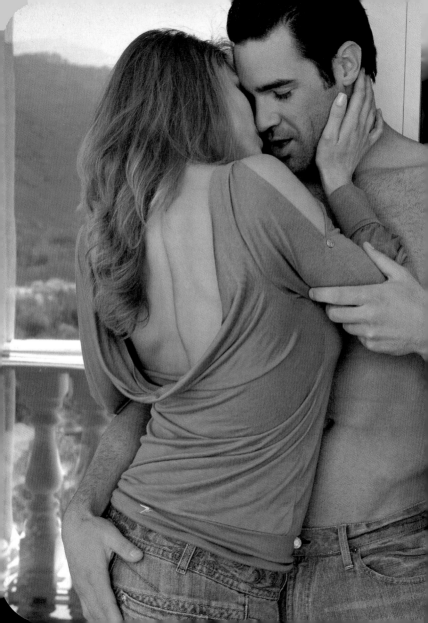

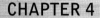

CHAPTER 4

My Right-Hand Man: Masturbatory Techniques

I believe every woman should have an orgasm a day. *Every* woman! *Every* day! Single, married, happily, or not. And she should own a veritable wardrobe of vibrators— sex life accessories. Isn't it time you got yours?

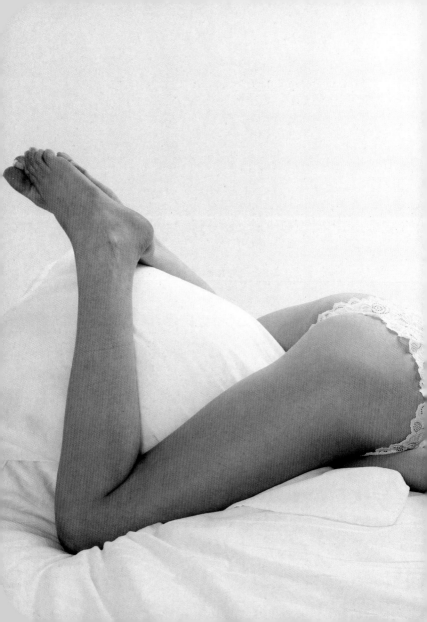

Why an orgasm a day? Orgasm is a great stress-reliever. It works naturally, like the progressive muscle-relaxation technique, which teaches stressed people to clench and release every muscle in their body.

In addition, orgasm can do the following:

- Relieve minor aches and pains, including headaches, by sending waves of endorphins—natural painkillers—throughout your body

- Help make you more comfortable with and knowledge-able about your body, which makes you more likely to orgasm with your partner

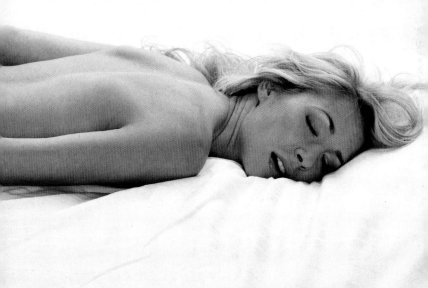

Why Vibrators?

For some women, the quickest way to an orgasm involves using a vibrator. Why do we like to play with vibrators? They're fun! It's all about the pleasure—and pleasure is a good thing, not only for selfish reasons. You're undoubtedly a nicer person when you're sexually satisfied.

Most vibrators are designed to stimulate the clitoris and are used externally. Some go inside, like dildos. Standard models get the job done, and quickly if you like. This is the vibe to use when you just need that O and don't have time for sensual or fantasy play. But you can also play as long as you want with them. Other models have more features.

If you are new to vibrators, here's a breakdown, including brand names of some of the best toys.

Hitachi Magic Wand

Often called "the Cadillac of vibrators," Hitachi is the largest-selling vibrator worldwide. It's also a large vibrator. Marketed as "a muscle massager," it's available in drugstores as well as sex toy shops.

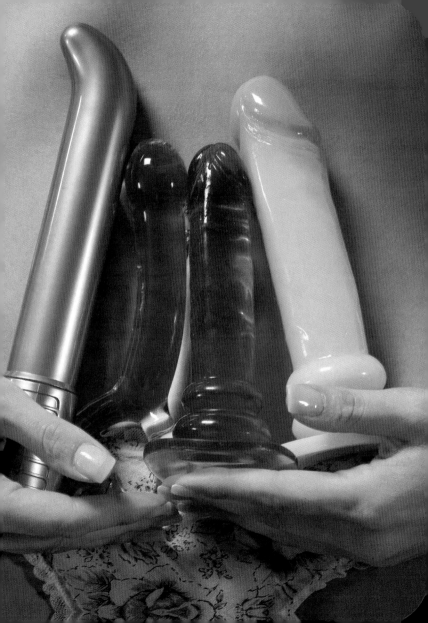

Eroscillator 2

The only sex toy endorsed by the legendary Dr. Ruth Westheimer, the Eroscillator resembles an electric toothbrush in size and shape. It oscillates rather than vibrates, so the motion is gentler against the clitoris but still effective.

Pocket Rocket

Tiny but powerful, this one stows away in a small handbag and gets the job done anywhere, anytime. You can change the texture of the vibe and the feeling of the vibrations by adding a jelly sleeve.

Fukuoku 9000

The top-of-the-line finger vibe, Fukuoku is a great couple's toy. Finger vibes wrap around or fit over your finger and are perfect for clitoral stimulation during intercourse. Finger Fun is a waterproof version.

SaSi

The "intelligent" vibe feels almost like a tongue—and remembers what you like. SaSi programs your responses for the next time.

The Butterfly

A strap-on vibrator, the Butterfly stimulates her clitoris during intercourse while giving him pleasurable sensations, too. The Sweetheart and many other vibes, some remote-controlled, work the same way.

G Swirl

Designed to hit the G-spot, this one and others like it are limited-use vibes. If G-spot orgasms are your thing, this is your toy. (You can also buy G-spot attachments for other vibes, including the Hitachi Magic Wand.)

The Rabbit

Ah, the Rabbit, with its multiple joys, is the choice when you have the time and inclination to indulge yourself. Insert the vibrating shaft so it hits your G-spot and let the ears of the rabbit riding the shaft tickle your clitoris as a vibrating band of pearls around the base stimulates your vaginal opening. Some Rabbits come without the pearls.

Laya Spot

One of the many new contour vibes, the Laya Spot is both chic and ergonomically correct. Designed to fit the curves of a woman's body, it is versatile and discreet.

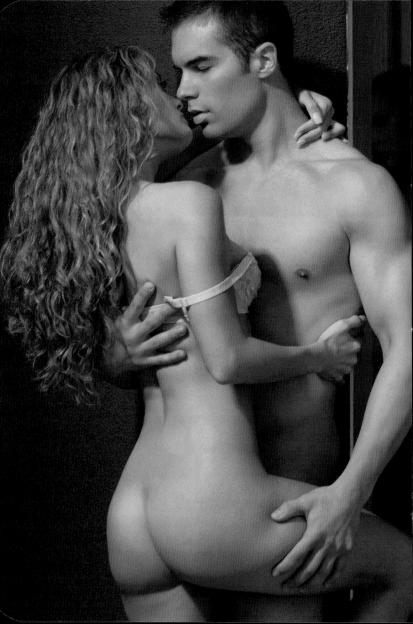

Talking Head

This Rabbit talks! The early version comes with computer chips—"lovers," like the French man and the girl who say what you want to hear. The latest version has an MP3 download, and you can program it with anything. On the horizon: an alliance with Clone-a-Willy that will produce a Talking Head shaped just like your guy and can speak in his voice.

OhMiBod

This is a slim wand that connects to an MP3 player all its own. Program your music into it and the wand vibrates to the beat. You can only find this one at Babeland—in stores or at babeland.com.

His Private Time

You don't have to tell most guys it's okay to masturbate. Unless they adhere to strict religious prohibitions, they aren't conflicted about giving self-pleasure, as many women still are.

Most women wonder if men can masturbate too much. You can do anything "too much" if that one activity is so obsessive that it prevents you from living a well-rounded life. But the odds are far greater that a man will be working rather than masturbating too much. When he's in a monogamous relationship where his libido runs hotter than hers, masturbation is a good thing. If she's complaining that they don't have sex often enough *and* he's masturbating a lot, he might not be a compulsive masturbator—but something's wrong somewhere.

But what if he is masturbating in front of the computer screen while she sleeps alone in their bed: Is something wrong with the relationship? Not necessarily. Don't be so quick to judge—and keep in mind that masturbation is a great learning tool.

Sex advisers are always telling women to masturbate so they will know how to reach orgasm. Men don't have a lot to learn in this regard: Friction equals orgasm. Most of the time, men masturbate quickly (and sometimes furtively). Take your time at it, and your sexual performance will improve.

The following techniques can be used to prolong masturbation and sex.

Edge Play

Continuously stimulate your penis to the point of impending ejaculation. Then stop. Yes, this takes some determination, but you can do it. Once your arousal level has subsided somewhat, stimulate continuously again to the point of impending ejaculation. Now stop. Repeat as

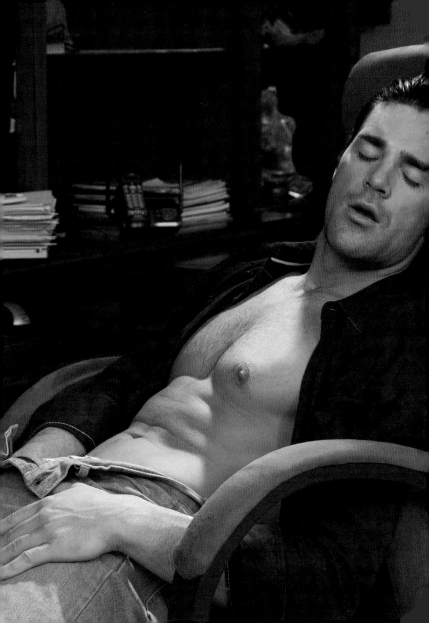

often as possible. Once you've learned how to prolong arousal during masturbation, you can transfer the skill to lovemaking.

Vary the Strokes

Most men masturbate in the same direct way, grasping the penis firmly and using a rapid up-and-down movement. That's why it's called "jerking off." Vary the strokes and the route is less direct. You gain more control over your orgasm. Try mixing in some of these strokes:

- **The Base Caress:** Slowly caress the base of your penis, squeezing the shaft and massaging the base.

- **The Slow Single Stroke:** Take your penis in one hand and stroke slowly up and down the shaft with your thumb or fingers from the other hand. Vary the pressure.

- **Circle Stroke:** Circle the head of your penis with the flat of your hand.

- **The Slow Two-Hand Stroke:** Use both hands on the shaft to perform the up-and-down stroke in slow motion.

- **The Cupped Hand:** Put the flat of one hand over the head of your penis. Use the fingers of the other hand to stroke the shaft. Vary the pressure and speed.

- **The Squeeze Stroke:** At the end of an up-down stroke, lightly squeeze the head of your penis.

- **The Open Hand Stroke:** Lay your penis in the palm of your hand and close your fingertips lightly around it. Use a slow, light stroke while keeping the hand open and fingers loosely curled around the penis. This feels more like a caress than a stroke and slows you down. It's the male masturbation version of "take the time to smell the roses."

His Toy: A Cock Ring

A plain cock ring fits around the base of the penis and over the balls to sustain his erection. Made from leather or metal, it keeps the blood flow in the penis, restricting the blood flow out—so it can't be worn for too long. Vibrating cock rings are generally made of softer material. They also fit around the base of the penis and over the balls, but not so tightly. The attached battery pack creates vibration that is exciting for him, and for her, too, if he wears it during intercourse.

Trojan now makes condoms with vibrating cock rings attached. Other manufacturers produce disposable vibrating cock rings. They don't have the power of the bigger toys, but they are more than a novelty. Chic women now carry them in their handbags . . . just in case.

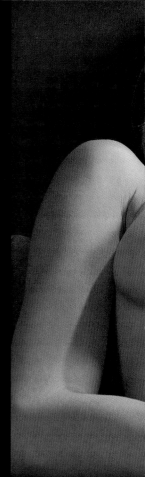

Mutual
Masturbation

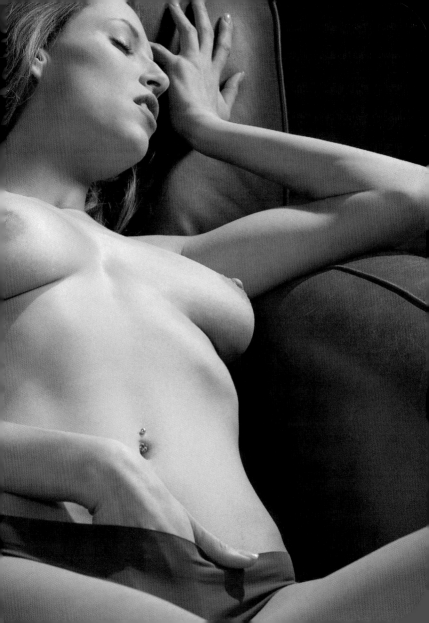

Mutual Masturbation

The Sexy Setup

If you're looking for a little fun and relaxation
(and perhaps a break from the demands of pleasuring
each other), this is the game for you. Tell your partner
you're going to share the pleasure tonight, but each
one of you controls your own destiny!

Rules & Tools

Create a seduction scene exactly as you would do for
"having sex": Dim the lights or light some candles and put
on some music. Arrange piles of pillows both for comfort
and good positions for watching each other get off.

Playing the Game

Sweet and safe: Feeling a little shy? Start by having
a glass of wine. Don't strip naked. Instead, don
an open shirt worn alone or thigh-highs, heels, and
a bustier. Start by flirting your way into it, as if you
and your partner were getting ready to be together.
Then slowly move off in your own direct, and relax

into the process. Close your eyes if you need to, then run your hands over your body the way you like to be touched. Fondle or squeeze your nipples, caress your thighs, and run your fingers lightly over your clitoris. Apply lubricant if needed and slowly circle your pubic mound, moving in to touch your clitoris and then moving away as if you're teasing yourself. Draw it out like this, pretending you're alone if you feel at all self-conscious. Chances are he's touching himself, too.

Hot and spicy: If you've played this game before, there are many ways to spice it up. Take turns masturbating—but stopping just before orgasm—then let your partner do the same. This kind of starting and stopping, all the while watching each other, can really prolong the pleasure—and heighten the orgasm. Alternatively, ask your partner to play a partial role, such as fondling your nipples from behind while you caress your clitoris. (Don't be surprised if he tries to slip his penis inside you once you've come!) If he likes it, stroke his nipples while he masturbates, nibble on his neck, lightly caress his lower back, or lick your way up his thighs. The combination of his own touch and your involvement is sure to send him over the edge.

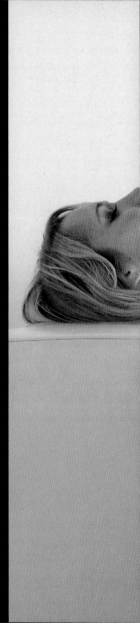

Masturbation Slave

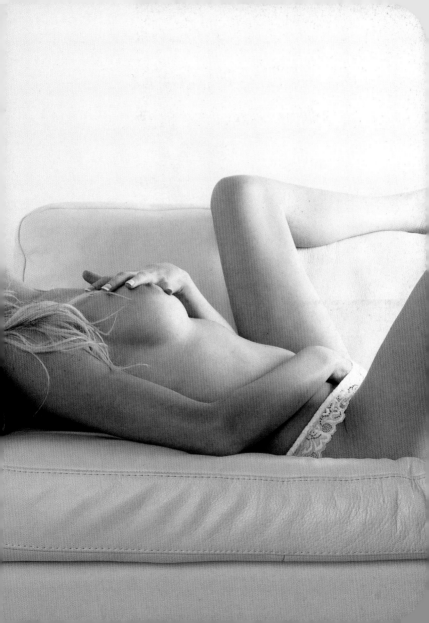

Masturbation Slave

The Sexy Setup

Tell your lover that you've got a game he's sure to love (especially if he likes being dominated). Tell him you're the beautiful Middle-Eastern princess, and he's the handsome masturbation slave who has to touch himself whenever his mistress desires.

Rules & Tools

Dress in your favorite Middle-Eastern princess outfit: Put on your sexiest bikini-style top, bikini bottoms, sheer skirt and a decorative belt, choker, and arm bands. Dress your lover in a loincloth or nothing at all. Assemble a pair of handcuffs, choker, or other props as desired.

Playing the Game

Sweet and safe: Order your lover to touch himself while you watch. If you want him to caress your breasts, suck your nipples, or squeeze your buttocks at the same time, order him to do so until you want him to stop. Don't let him orgasm—order him to stop from time to time, then mix in having him hand-feed you, massage your shoulders, or even watch a sexy movie together. Make him and start and stop masturbating at your whim—and tease him by masturbating yourself.

Hot and spicy: Buy your lover a choker and leash and lead him from room to room like a dog. When you want him to masturbate, tell him to do it (or face punishment). Keep a paddle or crop on hand for gently punishing his failure to use proper enthusiasm or for showing any sign of disrespect. Ready to really step it up a notch? Make your lover masturbate in a public place, such as a parked car or a spot in the woods, while you watch! Remember, you're in charge!

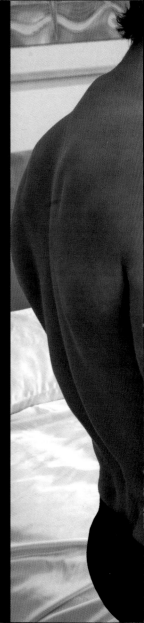

Learn His Strokes

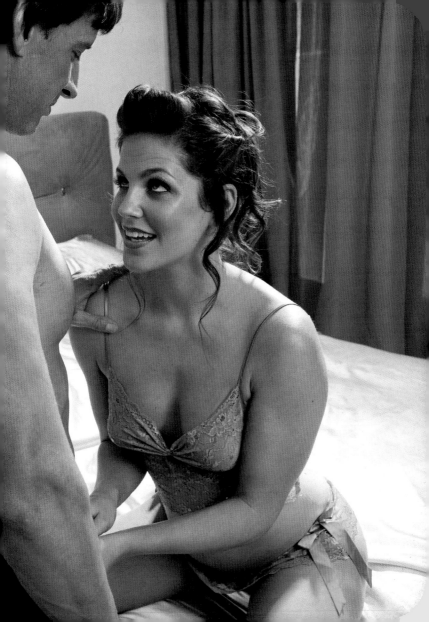

Learn His Strokes

The Sexy Setup

Most men masturbate in the same direct way, but this game involves you learning a variety of different strokes and testing which ones he likes best. Tell your lover you're ready for a "knowledge transfer" between his masturbatory hand and your hands, fingers, and palms.

Rules & Tools

Set a sexy scene, whether that means putting clean, silky sheets on the bed, setting up a soft rug in front of the fireplace, or lighting candles in your bathroom and getting into the tub together!

Playing the Game

Sweet and safe: Ask him to demonstrate each of the following techniques, then try to replicate the stroke yourself. Slowly caress the base of his penis, squeezing the shaft and massaging the base. Take his penis in one hand and stroke slowly up and down the shaft with your thumb or fingers from the other hand. Vary the pressure.

Circle the head of his penis with the flat of your hand, using any tiny drops of semen as lubrication while you rub your palm around. Use both hands on the shaft and perform the up-and-down stroke in slow motion.

Hot and spicy: Ready to take it up a notch? Put the flat of one hand over the head of his penis. Use the fingers of the other hand to stroke the shaft. Vary the pressure and speed—and ask him for verbal feedback. At the end of an up-down stroke, lightly squeeze the head of his penis while you kiss him deeply. Last but not least, lay his penis in the palm of your hand and close your fingertips lightly around it, using a slow, light stroke while keeping the hand open. This feels more like a caress than a stroke, and it slows him down. It's the male stroking version of "taking the time to smell the roses".

GAME 19

Door-to-Door Vibrator Salesman

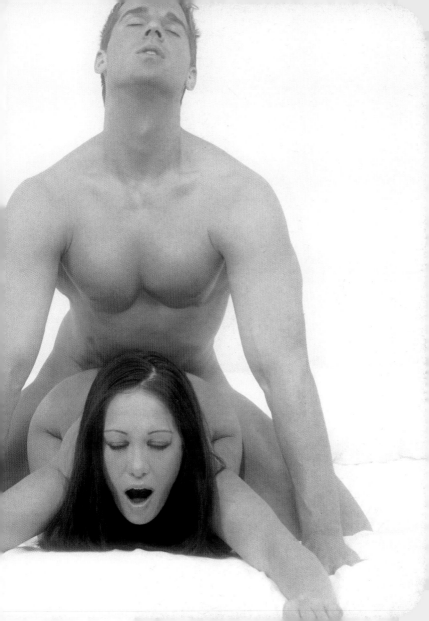

Door-to-Door Vibrator Salesman

The Sexy Setup

This fantasy game is purrrrrfect for men who like to role-play...and pull out all the toys! Just dress in a suit and pretend to be a door-to-door vibrator salesman. Try and surprise your lover when she thinks you're off at work or busy doing something else.

Rules & Tools

You'll need a suit, briefcase, pamphlets, and most important of all, a selection of vibrators.

Playing the Game

Sweet and safe: Ring the doorbell, then come into the house and explain that you have some very exciting products to show her. Take out the vibrators one by one, taking your time handling each one and explaining which are best suited for what types of play. Ask her if she'd like to borrow one and try it out (with you watching, of course)!

Hot and spicy: Come into the house and lay down the rules: You can only show her the products if she's naked, so the first thing she has to do is strip down (or get into something comfortable, like a short and sexy bathrobe). What's more, you're going to demonstrate their effectiveness on her, whether she likes it or not. At this point you can pull out some silk ties or handcuffs and bind her arms or legs to a chair leg. Then run through the product line one by one, taking as much time as you like to demonstrate just how effective the devices are for stimulation, teasing, and perhaps even orgasm. Ready to step it up a notch? Ask her swap roles and test the vibrators on you—perhaps you'd like to try anal stimulation!

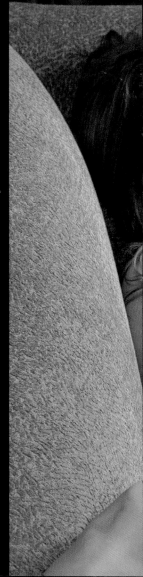

GAME 20

Finger Fun

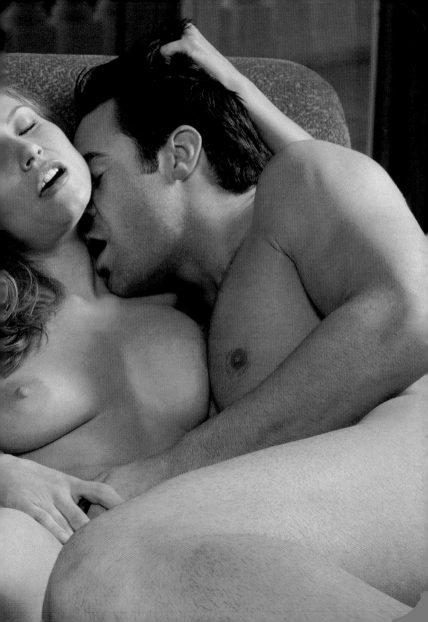

Finger Fun

The Sexy Setup

Call your lover and tell her you've got some fingers
that are itching to do some exploring and some toys
that will add to the fun. Remember to use her fingers
as well as yours!

Rules & Tools

You'll need an assortment of finger toys for this
game or a selection of miniature vibrators.

Playing the Game

Sweet and safe: Kiss your lover passionately, nuzzle
her neck, and slowly undress her with both hands. Have
her lie down or get comfortable in a sofa chair, then
start at her toes. Arming yourself with your finger toys
or miniature vibrators, tickle her every fantasy. Lick her
toes while you finger her labia, then move up to nibble
her thighs while she stimulates her clitoris. Have her

squeeze her own nipples while you add some tongue action, then move back to her masturbating and you using the finger toy on her nipples. She's sure to experience a mind-blowing orgasm!

Hot and spicy: Get your lover hot and wet, then ask her to kneel on all fours so you can enter her from behind. As you slowly penetrate her from behind, have her stimulate her clitoris using the finger vibrator. Try to time your climaxes together. Alternatively, have her use the finger vibrator on your nipples, perineum, or other hot spots while you masturbate to orgasm.

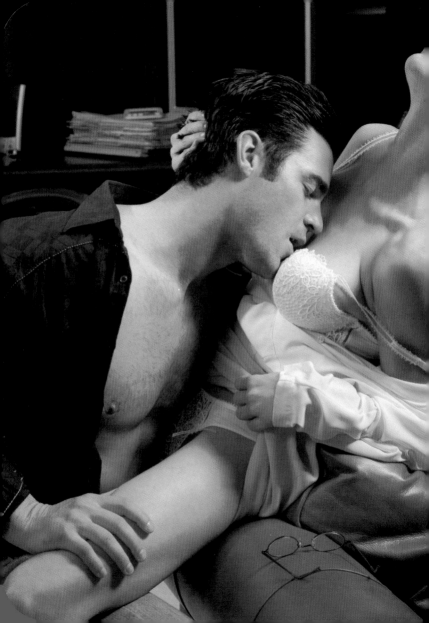

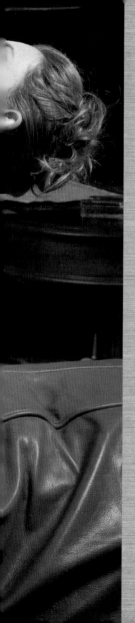

CHAPTER 5

Prime the Pump: Great Foreplay Techniques

Seduction is largely a mind game. If you play it well, your lover feels interesting and desirable. A truly seductive person is the man or woman you cannot own. He or she will share himself or herself with you, but not give it way. Now that is sexy.

Foreplay: Orgasm's Great Prelude

Sometimes a quickie is just what you want or need. You're both hot for one another because the foreplay has probably been going on in your minds for hours, maybe days. If she's savvy enough to masturbate a few minutes before the encounter, you will both likely reach orgasm.

Other times, a little to a lot more foreplay is required. And on special occasions, seduction and foreplay can be prolonged, or turned into erotic events that could almost stand on their own if you didn't want that orgasm so badly.

We all know the elements of foreplay, but they're worth repeating: Building on the sexual tension created by holding, touching, and caressing. Whispering endearments or naughty talk. Kissing. Sensual body stroking. Erotic massage (in longer periods of foreplay). Manual genital play. And let's not forget oral sex, which can also be an end in itself.

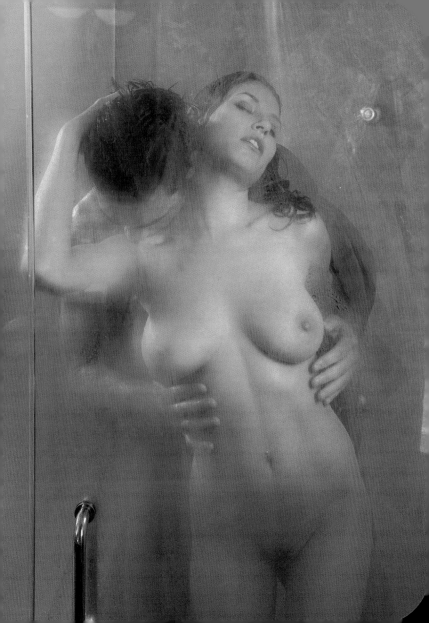

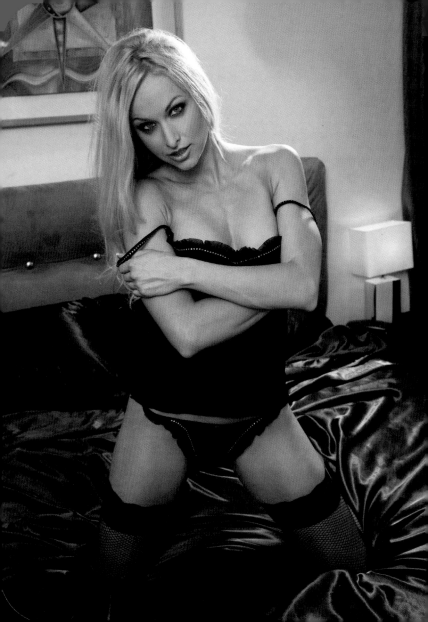

Step Up the Foreplay

A high state of arousal usually leads to a more powerful orgasm, so here are some techniques for moving your foreplay out of the ordinary!

Teasing

Teasing is seductive. It can be visual or verbal. Teasing plays with the mind, triggering fantasies, making promises you may or may not keep.

The Visual Tease

From little things like unbuttoning the first few buttons (his or hers) of your top or exposing the lacy tops of your thigh-high stockings when you cross your legs (generally her) to doing a slow strip for your lover, the visual tease is successful because both men and women are erotic visualizers.

Capitalize on this by "invitational dressing" when you go out. Some things always work: for her, high heels, cleavage, and the glimpse of firm nipples beneath a silk shirt; for him, a well-tailored suit, open dress shirt, with tie cast aside for the evening. Some things work only for you. Figure out what they are.

And don't forget this simple lesson: Learn how to walk. He strides smoothly and purposefully. She has a loose, undulating walk straight from the pelvis. Here's how to get that—and tickle that Kundalini energy.

- **The Pelvic Bounce:** Lie on a bed or the floor on your back with your palms on either side of your buttocks, knees bent. Lift your pelvis slightly and let it down, bouncing your lower back gently as you inhale sharply.

- **The Pelvic Thrust:** Stand with your hands on your hips. Move your pelvic area in a circular motion to the right, then to the left. Exhale as you thrust your pelvis forward in the motion. Inhale on the backward pull.

The Verbal Tease

Have you ever carried on an e-mail or text-message correspondence with a potential hot date, only to have your fantasies smashed merely by the sound of his or her voice?

Voice is important. Pitch your voice lower. Listen to how you sound on tape. If you have a nasal whine or a devastating accent issue, strive to change that.

Watch those sweet nothings and double entendres. They can sound shallow, foolish, or girlish/boyish. Verbal seduction is all about sounding desirable.

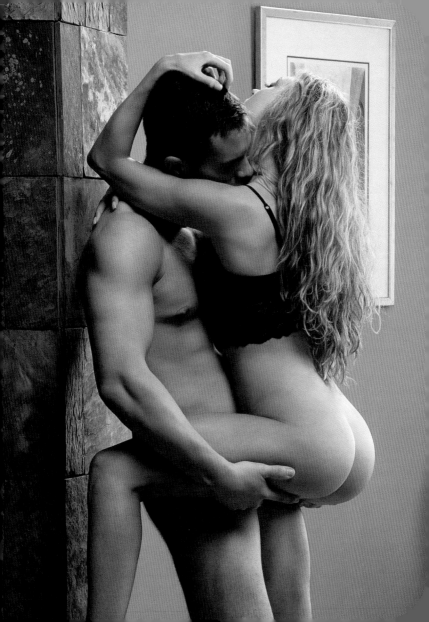

The Essential Kiss

If you don't like the way someone kisses or responds to your kisses, you're probably not going to find him or her to be an exceptional lover. The mouth is an erotic organ, visible, accessible, yet private. The kiss is important to men, but essential to women. Its power is so great that even scientists acknowledge the kiss is a form of personal chemistry, sending biological signals through the chemistry in our saliva. And too much saliva drowns a good kiss. Here's a few pointers for perfecting the art of kissing:

- Start kissing somewhere else and work your way up to her mouth. Nuzzle her neck, lick her ears, and kiss her throat.

- If you are naked in bed, kiss the backs of her knees. Lick her nipples. Alternate the rough side of your tongue (top) with the smooth side (bottom) for different sensations. (This works on men, too.)

- If you are fully clothed, kiss the back of her hand. Turn it over. Kiss her palm. Then let your lips rest on her wrist until you feel her pulse beating in your lips.

- Take her (or his) face in your hands. Brush your lips across hers lightly. Pull back. Put your lips on hers and press gently as you look into her eyes.

- Explore one lip at a time with light, playful, teasing kisses. Gently suck each lip. Run the tip of your tongue around its edges, inside and out.

- Now French kiss. With the tip of your tongue, play with her tongue, the inside of her lips, the edges of her teeth. Kiss her passionately, but don't assault her mouth with your tongue.

Touching and Stroking

What is the first physical connection you have with a lover? You touch one another's hands or arms during conversation. Maybe she straightens his tie. He brushes the hair back off her face. If the hands feel right on the other's flesh, the touches escalate. But if they don't, it all ends there.

Touch is a key element of lovemaking, yet few of us work on our hand skills once we get past the point of having our touch accepted by the new lover.

First, get the touch right. When you are holding your lover and caressing her (or him), touch her the way she likes to be touched. Most people respond to light caresses, with the pressure escalating as the excitement builds. Don't go straight for breasts or genitals. Stroke her collarbone. Rub his chest. Fondle thighs and buttocks. When you are naked, add some unexpected touches, such as the following:

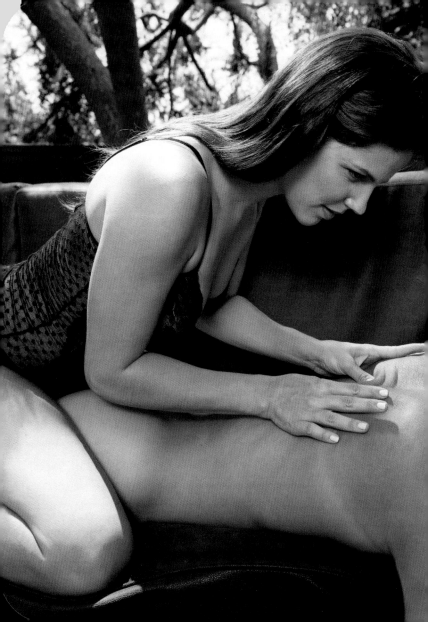

- Warm up to sexual touch with light and playful massage—a good starting point is to approach your lover from behind and massage his or her shoulders.

- Use the pads of your fingers to play lightly over your lover's body.

- Try "scent kissing," or inhaling the scent of his or her body in places like the nape of the neck, breasts, and inner thighs.

- Use feathers, silk, rose petals, or other materials to stroke or tease nipples and genitals.

- Caress his penis between your breasts.

- Use a fingernail to bring out the goose bumps on your lover's buttocks, lower back, or belly.

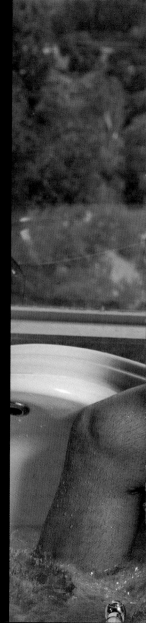

Queen of Foreplay

(Hands-on Foreplay for Her)

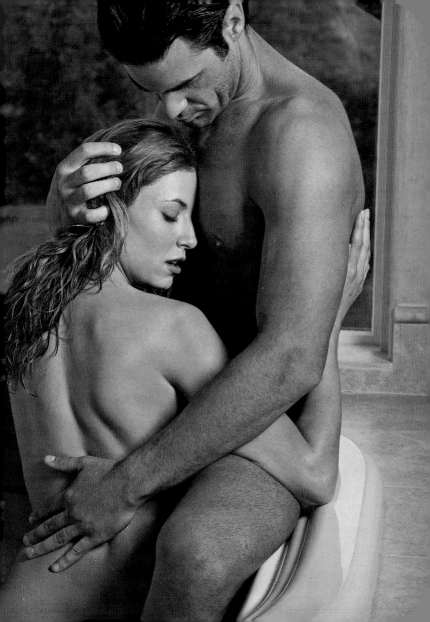

Queen of Foreplay

(Hands-on Foreplay for Her)

The Sexy Setup

Here's a game where she gets to be queen—and you're the prince who's come to charm her with your spectacular foreplay techniques.

Rules & Tools

Set a sensual scene for your encounter. Leave the sex toys in the drawer for tonight and focus on using just your own mouth and hands to drive her crazy with desire.

Playing the Game

Sweet and safe: Take her face in your hands, kiss her eyelids, and, with one hand still holding her face, stroke her cheeks and forehead with your thumb. As you kiss her mouth or neck, massage her breasts with the flat of your hand, then slip off her blouse and bra in a slow, sensual movement. Once her breasts are bare, glide your hand, with the first two fingers open in a V, up each of her breasts, catching her nipple in the V. Now kiss that nipple. Take her nipple *gently* between two fingers and pinch. Slip off her remaining clothes, caress her inner thighs from her knees up. Let your thumb or fingers graze her vulva as you reach the top of her thighs. Don't forget to caress her back, shoulders, legs and belly. Is she moaning with desire?

Hot and spicy: Use light circular motions with your fingertips on her genital area. Part her labia and make long strokes on the outside lips. Then curve one or two fingers and use the space between the knuckle and joint to massage her inner and outer lips lightly in a back-and-forth motion. Alternate that stroke with one using your thumb or first finger alone. Rotate your fingers around her clitoris, alternating a clockwise and counterclockwise motion. Stroke down with one finger on either side of her clitoris, rotate, and stroke down again. If she likes direct clitoral stimulation, take the clitoris between two fingers and gently rotate. But if, like many women, she can't stand the intensity of that stroke, circle your fingertips above the clitoris (at the twelve o'clock point). Ready for more? Add the G-spot stroke. While continuing the twelve o'clock rotation on her clitoris, insert a finger or two into her vagina and massage her G-spot. Continue to stroke her clitoris as you massage her G-spot, and don't be surprised if she ejaculates during this mind-blowing orgasm.

King of Foreplay

(Hands-on Foreplay for Him)

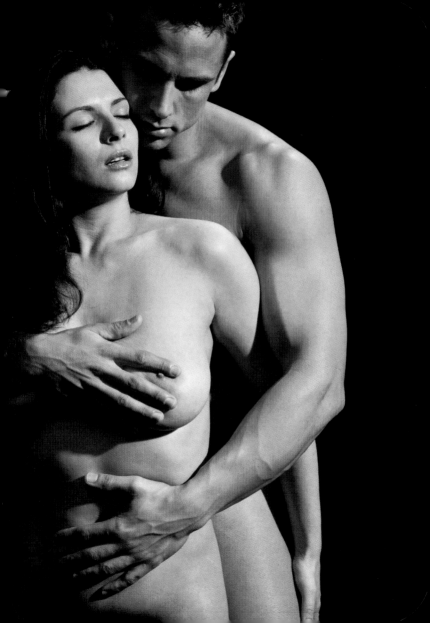

King of Foreplay

(Hands-on Foreplay for Him)

The Sexy Setup

Here's a chance to pay back your lover for all the wonderful things he's done for you. Text him a flirty message telling him he's king for the day and you're a subject in his court who's dying to practice some newfound foreplay techniques. Chances are just the message will get him hard!

Rules & Tools

Create a lusty lair with soft blankets, animal rugs, or other sensual fabrics. Put on some soft music, light a few candles, and open a bottle of wine. If desired, use your imagination and dress like a subject in King Henry the Eighth's lusty court: Cleavage is a must, and perhaps a long skirt with no underwear underneath!

Playing the Game

Sweet and safe: Knead his shoulders and back very gently to help him relax. Make circular motions with your hands on his back from the spine upward and to the sides of his body. Alternate the circular motions with smooth, gliding strokes. Remove his shirt as you kiss the nape of his neck, then slowly remove his pants and underwear. Try single- or two-finger gliding strokes on his inner thighs, back, and the sides of his neck, then repeat the long, gliding strokes on his chest, stomach, and thighs. Do something entirely unexpected: Use the single-finger stroke on his face and the delicate areas around his eyelids and ears. Run your finger along his throat as you kiss him deep and hard to along the base of his neck and down his chest. Ready to step it up? Move on to hot and spicy.

Hot and spicy: Kneel between his legs, occasionally kissing or stroking his inner thighs. Take his testicles one at a time very gently between your fingers and thumb, then hold a testicle in the palm of your hand and tickle it lightly with the pads of your fingers. If he likes it, repeat on the other side. If he's not comfortable, move on to his golden shaft. Hold the base of his penis in one hand and work your other hand in a circular, upwardly twist-ing movement to the head. Use the palm of that hand to caress the head of his penis. Take his penis in both hands. Imagine building a fire with his penis as the stick: Using a rolling/rubbing motion, starting at the base. Roll/rub up to the head, keeping his penis between your palms. Use only upward motions. Start over at the base when you reach the head. Start slowly. Increase the speed as he gets closer to orgasm. Lean forward so that he ejaculates onto your breasts!

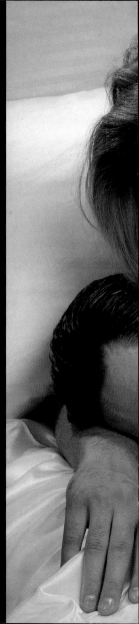

GAME 23

Reviving a Fallen Soldier

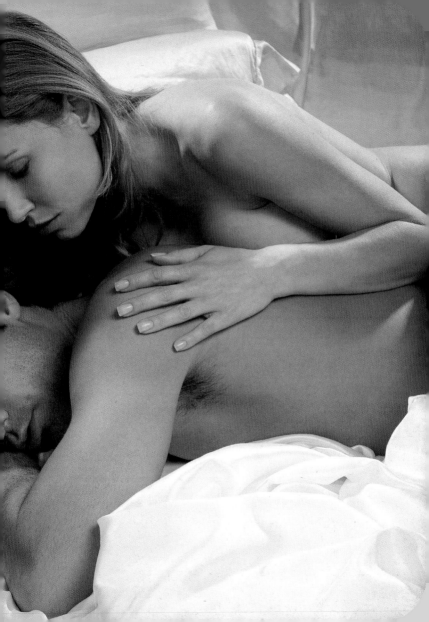

Reviving a Fallen Soldier

The Sexy Setup

Every man, at some time or another, has lost his erection.
No worries—just use one of the techniques outlined to
turn his game back on!

Rules & Tools

Rule number one: Don't make a big deal of it, and don't
take it personally. Instead, go with the flow—and remind
him how you love being with him, regardless of whether
his solider is ready for battle!

Playing the Game

Sweet and safe: Ask him to focus on you for awhile.
Have him kiss, caress, stroke, and fondle you—or even
give you orgasm using his tongue. Chances are he'll have
an erection after that, but if not, move on to the Cowgirl
in Charge. First, straddle him. Grasp the base of his penis
firmly in one hand. Use the head of his penis to stroke your
vulva and clitoris. When you are ready, lower yourself
onto his penis without letting go of the base. Grasp the
first third of his penis in your strong PC muscle. Simulate
thrusting with that muscle. (This alone may revive his

erection.) Lean forward, supporting yourself on one hand resting beside his body. (Your other hand still has that penis. Don't let go of it.) Work his penis up and down with your hand and PC muscle. Alternate that with "thrusting of the head" stroke, or using the head of his penis against your clitoris.

Hot and spicy: Sometimes even a good blow job or your best hand job may not be enough to revive a fallen solider. The Stand Up Kiss, works by combining the two. Start by holding his penis firmly in one hand. Take it into your mouth, moving the top third of the shaft in and out. Use the fingers of your other hand to stroke his perineum in a light, ticking fashion. If he responds to gentle scratching, do that. When he becomes erect, use one hand to do a circular twisting motion up the shaft. Then start at the bottom again. At the same time you're twisting up, swirl your tongue around the corona. Alternate the swirl with the butterfly flick—flicking your tongue rapidly across the corona. Continue the hand move while taking his testicles into your mouth, one at a time, and sucking lightly. Flick your tongue rapidly across his perineum. Go back to the head of his penis and alternate swirling, flicking, and sucking. Remember: Don't take his penis too far into your mouth when you suck or you won't be able to pull off the suction.

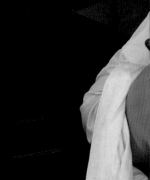

GAME 24

Preheat the Oven

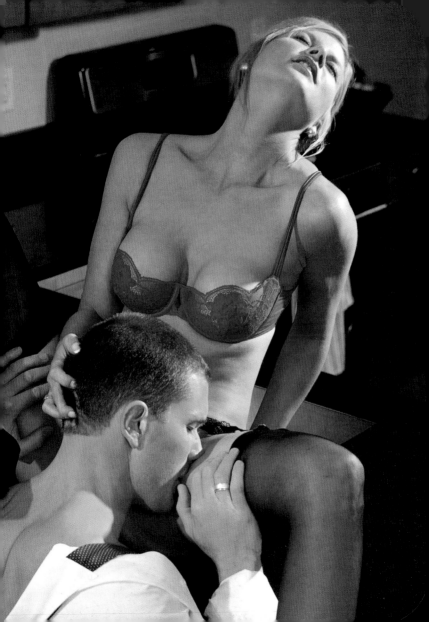

Preheat the Oven

The Sexy Setup

Put away the pots and pans—you'll want to play this racy game of foreplay right on the kitchen counter! Tell your lover that your oven needs preheating. What's more, your drawers are open and you're serving something hot and spicy for dinner.

Rules & Tools

Clean off the counters and dim the lights. Wear an apron with nothing under it and line up some sexy kitchen tools or gadgets, such as a soft pastry brush or a pair of tongs (if you like it a little rougher). Set the timer to however long you want the foreplay to last.

Playing the Game

Sweet and safe: Position yourself on the counter, then ask him to remove your apron using his teeth. Once you're naked, ask him to prepare you for higher temperatures by rubbing you down with massage oil. Make sure he spends ample time on your breasts, rump, and inner thighs. Ready to step it up a notch?

Ask your lover to blindfold you with a kitchen towel and turn you on using his choice of kitchen utensils. Have him tickle your inner thighs or genitals with a soft pastry brush, gently pinch your nipples with tongs, blow cool air on your neckline using a turkey baster, and so forth.

Hot and spicy: Lie on the counter, let your lover blindfold you with a kitchen towel, and ask him to bring out the tray of ice cubes. Start by passing an ice cube back and forth between you while you kiss. Have him hold the cube in his mouth while he explores your body, alternating between an icy tongue and hot breath. The goal: Melt all the ice cubes in the tray. Alternatively, have him lie on the counter and play "heat and ice." While performing fellatio, vary the temperature of your mouth. Start with normal body temperature. Then, using your hand to stimulate his penis, fill your mouth with ice cubes. Wait until your tongue is numb before spitting out the ice. Apply your frozen tongue to his penis. This feels like a jolt of sexual electricity. After a few minutes, when you oral temperature is back to normal, repeat the procedure, this time filling your mouth with a hot liquid. His orgasm is more intense after playing with heat and ice!

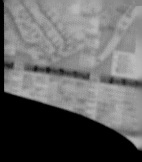

Variations on a Theme: Public Foreplay

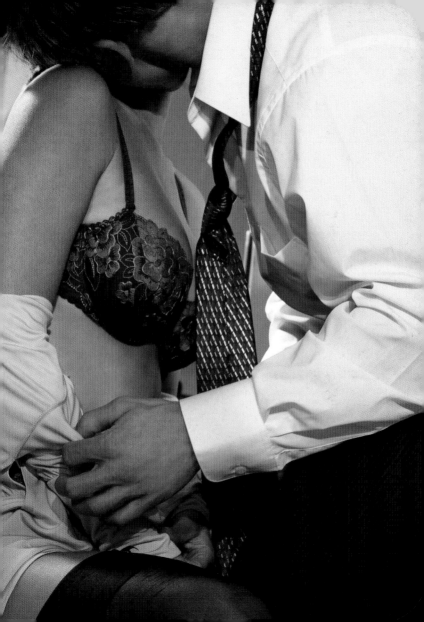

Variations on a Theme: Public Foreplay

The Sexy Setup

You've seen that couple who can't keep their hands off each other in a restaurant, at a party, anywhere in public. Maybe you've *been* that couple. This game is all about trying on different flavors of foreplay, but all of them should take place in public!

Rules & Tools

There's really only one rule here: Don't let your foreplay get out of hand! The goal is to build the tension—and save the release for later, perhaps at home or at the hotel. If you absolutely can't control your passion and you find yourself needing to come in public, just remember not to get caught—being naked in public can be against the law. (On the flip side, the thrill of playing but not getting caught may make your public foreplay even hotter!)

Playing the Game

Sweet and safe: Pick a dark booth in your neighborhood bar. Kick off your shoe and play with his leg—all the way up his leg. Alternatively, sit on his lap on a park bench and make out, or kiss and fondle one another on the beach at night. Ready to step it up a notch? Consider car sex! You don't have to park on a lover's lane, either—the driveway or garage will do. Part of the thrill in this game is the limited range of motion. The space is tight—and that feels illicit—so try these moves on for size: Push the frontseats as far forward as they go, ask him to lie down on the backseat, and ride him like a cowgirl (with your clothes on!). Have your lover kneel with one leg on each front seat and push his penis toward you over the armrest. You sit in the backseat and suck him (but don't let him come!). Last but not least, get out of the car, sit on the hood, and have him explore your clitoris with his tongue!

Hot and spicy: Try a game of "ride and tease" on the elevator at work, in a department store, or at the airport. The goal? Tease each other between floors so that once you get home (or back to his office), you can have hot and steamy intercourse. Start the game by getting on the elevator together, push the button for every single

(continued on page 188)

floor, and stand at the back. If no one else gets on, kiss, fondle, and touch each other as much as possible before the elevator stops at the next floor and the doors open. If other people are in front of you, discreetly fondle his crotch or let him grab your behind until you're alone again. As the doors open and close, continue this teasing action to build the excitement. Once you reach the top floor, repeat the game on the way down. Better yet, find a hidden stairwell, put one leg up on the railing, and let him enter you standing up to release the pent-up tension!

MORE SEXY FOREPLAY IDEAS

Try these on for size, but only if you can carry them off in the spirit of fun:

- Send naughty text messages to one another.

- When you dress to leave, "forget" your panties or briefs.

- Apply an erotic temporary tattoo to your body— and make him or her find it.

- Eat off one another's naked bodies.

- Find sexy adult games online and play them.

- Play Strip Anything. (It doesn't have to be poker.)

- Assign some sex acts as "rewards" or "punishments" for losing at tennis, being late for a dinner date, and so on.

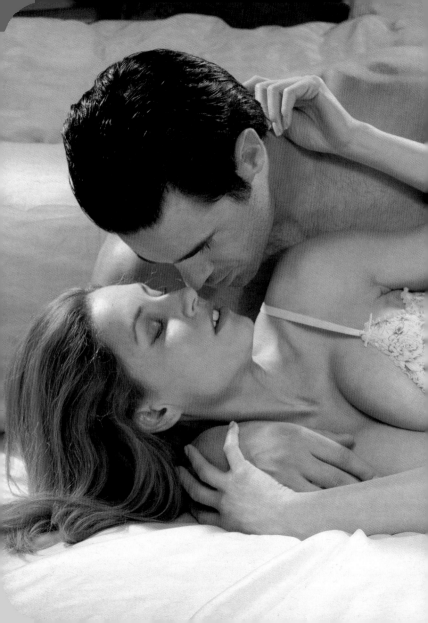

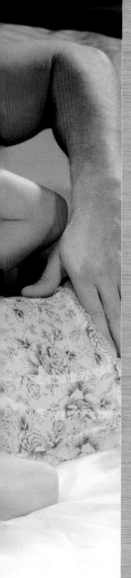

CHAPTER 6

His and Her Orgasms

Are you ready to come now? So ready that you're impatient for the instant gratification formula? If you're a woman and you have trouble reaching orgasm, you will learn how to get there more reliably and in less time by reading this chapter. If you're a man who wants stronger, longer orgasms, you can get those, too.

Her Orgasms

There are many techniques for reaching orgasm more reliably and in less time.

And there are a lot of theories—many conflicting—about orgasm, mostly female orgasm on how she can come and why she doesn't. Sexual response varies so much from one person to another and in every individual from one partner or situation to another that no answer applies universally. Other physical factors—everything from mild allergies to heart disease—also affects sexual response. What worked yesterday may not work today.

That said, you can find something here that will work. Play around with techniques until you find the right combination for you. The female orgasm is not elusive. It's right beneath your fingertips.

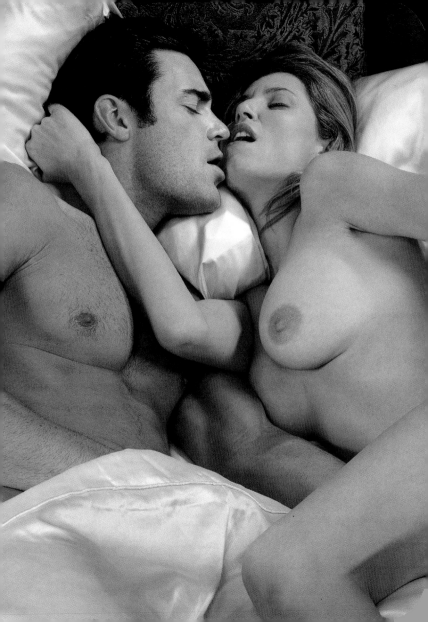

Why Orgasm?

Biologically speaking, the answer is simple for his orgasm: procreation. He has an orgasm and ejaculates, sending his sperm out to meet their fate. But women don't need an orgasm to fertilize eggs—so why (in the biological sense) do we have them at all?

Until very recently, the prevailing theory was that female orgasm somehow offered an evolutionary advantage. Scientists assumed a link between orgasm and reproductive success, positing, for example, that orgasm aided fertilization by helping draw sperm up through the cervix and into the uterus. A dissenting opinion, first expressed by anthropologist Donald Symons in 1979, was not popular. He concluded that female orgasm was simply a by-product of male orgasm (because both sexes develop from a common embryo plan). In other words, orgasm is only possible in women because it's necessary in men. Needless to say, scientists didn't like that, and neither did feminists!

Elizabeth Lloyd's 2006 book, *The Case of the Female Orgasm,* is an erudite and enlightened argument against all the adaptive biology theories. Yes, female orgasm is a by-product, she says, and not necessary to the procreation of the species. But the clitoris and sexual pleasure do serve an evolutionary purpose: They encourage women to have sex and thus get pregnant.

What Is an Orgasm?

In lay terms, an orgasm is generally defined as an intense, pleasurable response to genital stimulation, a release of sexual tension marked by a series of genital contractions, and the release throughout the body of natural chemicals that create feelings of euphoria and attachment. Scientists say it a bit differently, but one thing's for sure—it feels good!

Understanding why it feels so good isn't rocket science. When a woman is aroused, blood flow increases to the vagina, swelling the inner and outer lips and the clitoris. With enough intense physical and psychological stimulation, she will reach climax, during which the vagina, sphincter, and uterus contract simultaneously, and the blood congested in the vaginal area suddenly rushes back to the rest of the body. And that expulsion of tension and blood flow feels good!

Chemicals released in the brain do the rest of the feel-good work. Endorphins ease pain and elevate the sense of overall well-being. Oxytocin encourages those warm feelings of affection for her partner in orgasm. (And no big surprise: Women produce more oxytocin, or the "cuddly chemical," than men do.)

That chemical cocktail is most potent in the early stages of a relationship. It's called New Relationship Energy, or NRE. Lasting anywhere from eighteen

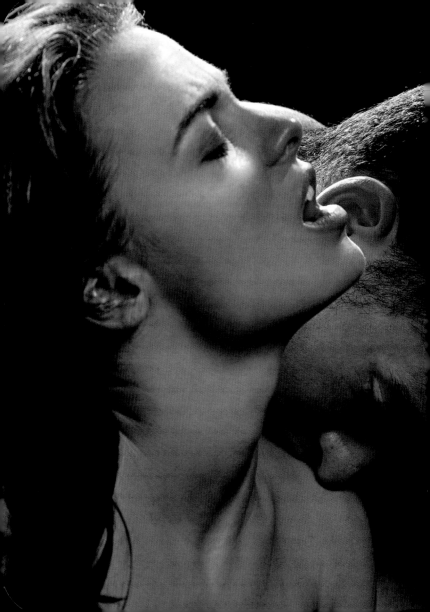

months to three years, NRE propels us into commitment, monogamy, and marriage—life choices we may begin to question when the drug wears off.

Nan Wise, neuroscience researcher, has developed a tool for understanding and managing desire: the Desire Curve. We all have a Desire Set Point, the level of sexual craving we naturally feel whether in a relationship or not. In a new relationship, the level curves up for eighteen months and reaches a plateau, where it stays for three years. Wise calls this period New Relationship Euphoria, or NREU. From the high, we all go back to the Desire Set Point. (In other words, hot monogamy is a lie.) Some people dip past the set point into Low Desire Syndrome —perhaps a by-product of misunderstanding.

Sexually skilled lovers, however, can manage their Desire Curves by creating peaks in the valleys of their set points. For them, intersecting Desire Curves can rise and fall like waves.

What Are the Kinds of Orgasm?

For many decades, female orgasm was defined as either/ or: clitoral or vaginal.

In 1953, Alfred Kinsey published a landmark study, *Sexual Behavior in the Human Female,* proclaiming that all female orgasms were achieved by clitoral stimulation, either direct or indirect. His findings were endorsed a decade later by pioneer sex researchers William Masters and Virginia Johnson, who isolated the orgasm in the lab and measured and quantified the process. The clitoral orgasm theory became the prevailing opinion among sex therapists until 1980, when Beverly Whipple and John Perry claimed their research proved the existence of the G-spot, putting the origin for the female orgasm back inside the vagina.

The G-spot theory is not uniformly accepted. The late Helen Singer Kaplan, Ph.D., a pioneer in sex therapy and founder of the nation's first clinic for sexual disorders, insisted that 75 percent of women do not reach orgasm without some kind of direct clitoral stimulation. Many studies in scientific journals have consistently reported that 60 to 75 percent of women do not reach orgasm without clitoral stimulation, with less than 10 percent of women reporting in most studies that they could, in fact, find their G-spots.

What can we learn from all this? Kinsey and Masters and Johnson did women a great service in promoting the power of the clitoris. And if you can find your G-spot, enjoy it. If you can't, *c'est la vie.*

A popular theory among sex authorities now is that women can reach orgasm in a variety of ways. Try them all and see what works for you. But remember: There is no right or wrong way to come.

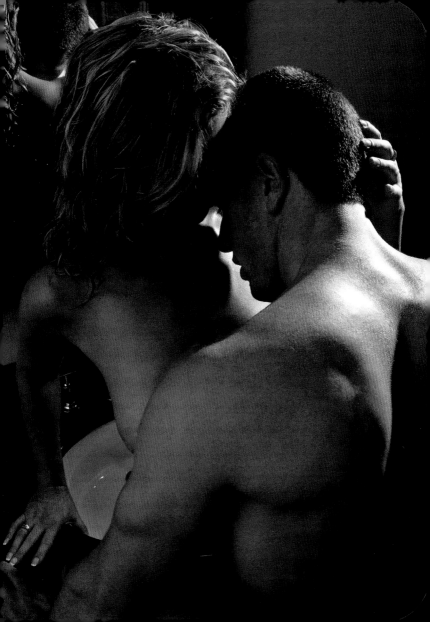

The orgasm routes are as follows:

Clitoral

The clitoris is rich in nerve endings, with more of them concentrated in that little organ than in the male penis. The clitoris is the only part of the body, male or female, designed purely for pleasure. Yes, the overwhelming majority of women do have clitoral orgasms.

Vaginal/Cervix

Every woman seems to want the vaginal orgasm achieved through penile thrusting alone. It is more likely to happen in two positions: on top and rear entry. You are more likely to experience vaginal/cervix orgasm if you don't begin intercourse until you are on the point of orgasm and you use your PC muscle while he's thrusting.

Vaginal/G-Spot

First, try to reach orgasm with a G-spot vibrator. That will show you where your G-spot is and how much stimulation it needs for orgasm. During intercourse, get into the woman-on-top position and lean back. Experiment with different angles until you feel that G-spot responding. (And play with your clitoris if you aren't getting what you need from the G-spot.)

Anal

Anal play is highly pleasurable for many women (and men), and some women do reach orgasm this way. The secrets to satisfaction? Your lover should spend a lot of time relaxing the anus and use lots of lube! (See Chapter 8 for more information.)

Extra-Genital

Some women can reach orgasm simply by having their breasts or nipples or inner thighs or other sensitive areas stimulated. This is most likely to happen after she has reached orgasm via other routes. Here are some techniques for making this happen:

- After she's had at least one orgasm, caress her vagina and perform cunnilingus if she requests it.

- When she is on the verge of another orgasm, move your hands and mouth away from her genitals. Stroke her breasts, nipples, inner thighs—whatever nongenital area she wants touched, kissed, or licked. She may be in such a state of hypersensitivity that she reaches orgasm this way, and the orgasm will feel like it is spread throughout her body.

- If not, stimulate her clitoris orally or manually as you continue to pay attention to nongenital areas.

Blended

Some women say that their best orgasms come when two areas are being stimulated simultaneously, for example, the clitoris and vagina or anus. It's possible that some orgasms reported as vaginal or anal are really blended. If you're stroking your clitoris while you're coming from another form of stimulation, it's a blended orgasm. (See Chapter 9 for more information.)

Why Do Some Women Come More Easily Than Others?

"More easily" usually means that women come during intercourse alone, because almost all women come during masturbation. The ability—or luck—to do that is rare enough to qualify as "not the norm," yet we continue to hold up the model of female orgasm via intercourse alone as the "norm" or "ideal." That isn't fair to women or to men who blame themselves for not being able to "make" her come.

Theories about why some women orgasm more easily than others usually come down to these two: She has a larger than average clitoris or, more likely, she has more extensive tangle of clitorial nerve endings, making it more likely that she gets the clitoral stimulation she needs for orgasm during intercourse alone.

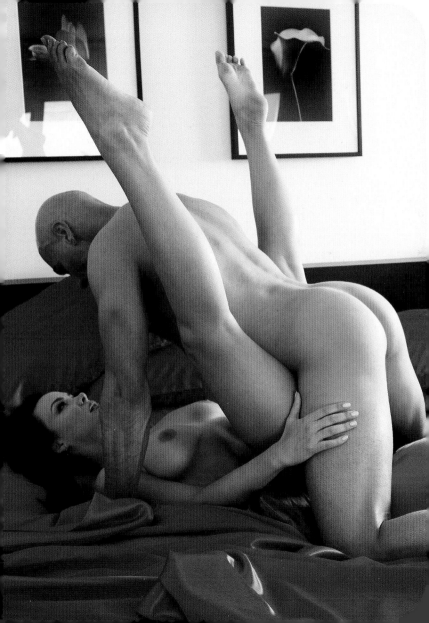

From my own extensive interviews of thousands of women over two decades, I believe that location, location, location is the answer. (However, many women who say they have a large or prominent clitoris also say they cannot come during intercourse alone.) Think of the clitoris as real estate you inherited.

A Word About Faking It

The advice to "fake it" may be the common wisdom, but it's terrible advice. Statistics from women's magazine surveys to research conduced by university psychology departments report that women do fake orgasm, and in consistently high numbers. Would you believe that 85 percent of women have faked an orgasm at least once in their lives? (And the other 15 percent are either virgins or liars.)

The biggest reason not to fake it is, you're saying, "Honey, *that* worked!" But it didn't. It won't work next time, either. Faking may end the sex, but it isn't going to make you happy.

I am not encouraging you to criticize his technique or blame him for not pleasing you. Ask for what you want and need in the moment, not later. Learn how to have an orgasm. And then make sure you do have them.

His Orgasms

The male orgasm has not received the same level of attention that the female orgasm has. Your local bookstore may have a couple dozen books on her orgasm and maybe one on his—and that will probably be a book about how he can come without ejaculating using Eastern erotic techniques. Orgasm is no problem for men, right? One orgasm is just as good as another for him, right? On the other hand, he doesn't have the unlimited orgasmic potential that she has, right?

While *having* an orgasm may not be the issue for him as it is for her, he does experience some orgasms as "better" than others. He can learn how to have more of those if he wants to do that. The potential for enriching his entire sexual experience through developing new orgasm skills is real.

How Does His Orgasm Differ from Hers?

Male orgasm is defined as the release of tension caused by the engorgement of blood in the genitals by contractions experienced in the penis and surrounding area, similar in timing, sequence, and length to the female orgasm. The big difference between his and hers

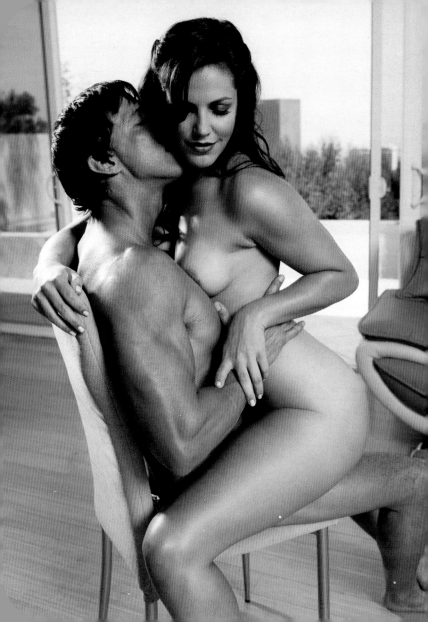

is that the male orgasm is considered "inevitable" while the female version is described as "elusive" or "problematic." His orgasm is "inevitable" for two reasons: Male masturbation is more acceptable than is female masturbation, and our model of partner sex is intercourse. Men reach orgasm by friction (penile thrusting) applied to the penis. While a man may achieve orgasm more reliably than his woman does, he doesn't have as many potential paths to ecstasy as are available to her.

Generally, men reach orgasm via stimulation of the head of the penis during intercourse or the up-and-down movement of the shaft during masturbation. There is more than one way to bring a penis to orgasm, however, including fellatio, manual stimulation, intercourse, anal play, and stimulating his P zone (perineum). As for a male G-spot, yes, he has one. See 17 for directions on how to find it.

If a man comes just by looking at a naked woman or holding and kissing her, he's fourteen (and way too young for her!) or suffers from premature ejaculation. While it's a good thing if a woman can come via extragenital stimulation, it's not so good if a man does. Thus, males orgasms are considered to be limited to three categories—ejaculatory, nonejaculatory, and multiple—with many experts discounting the possibility of nonejaculatory orgasm.

Can Men Have Multiples?

Whether or not men can have multiple orgasms depends largely on whether or not you accept that a man can have a nonejaculatory orgasm. Everyone acknowledges that a man does have a refractory period after ejaculation. Some men (especially, but not only, younger men) can become erect again in a short period of time and have another ejaculatory orgasm during one lovemaking session, but this is not defined as a multiple orgasm. Sexologists are not in agreement, however, on whether or not it is possible for him to experience the contractions of orgasm without ejaculation.

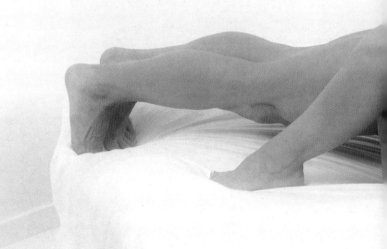

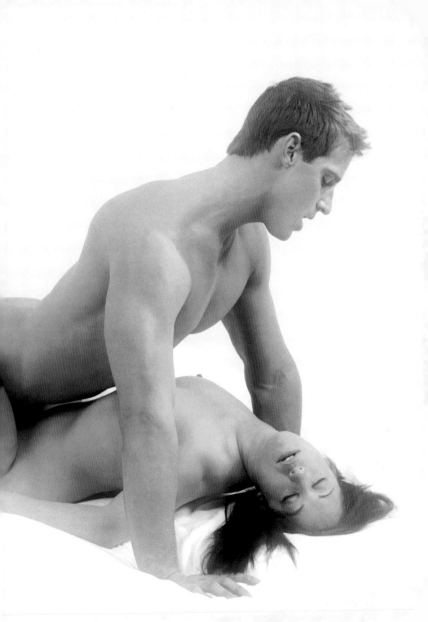

The guru of self-help books and workshops on male multiples is Stan Dale, who has a doctorate in human sexuality from the Institute for the Advanced Study of Sexuality in San Francisco. According to Dale, men can *learn* how to experience orgasm without ejaculation. His techniques for doing that rely heavily on mental control, something men under thirty-five or forty may not have. His main advice on the technique is to strengthen the PC muscle by doing Kegels (see 59) and to try to hold back ejaculation by using that muscle and telling yourself, "Not now, maybe later, but not now."

Repeatedly using the techniques for delaying ejaculation explained in the following section may be more effective. Some men do report that they can learn how to experience orgasmic contractions without ejaculation through repeated delaying maneuvers. Is the quest for orgasm without ejaculation worth the effort? You be the judge of that for yourself.

Delaying His Orgasm

The Eastern lovemaking arts emphasize delaying his ejaculation while intensifying her arousal. The goal is to bring her to orgasm during intercourse. As we've already figured out, he—and she—can make that happen by stimulating her clitoris. Many men do want to sustain their erections for longer periods of time during intercourse for other reasons, such as extending the pleasure for him and his partner. Here are a few techniques.

The Three-Finger Draw

Practiced in China for five thousand years, this technique is simple and—men tell me—effective. Locate the midpoint of your perineum, that sensitive area between the base of the testicles and the anus. Using the three longest fingers of your right hand, apply pressure—not too light and not too hard—to this spot as soon as you feel the inevitability of orgasm. Your fingers should be curved slightly. The trick is in finding the right spot and applying the pressure in the nick of time.
That may take a little practice.

The Big Draw

This one requires a strong PC muscle (see 59). When you feel ejaculation is imminent, stop thrusting. Pull back to approximately 1 inch of penetration, but don't withdraw completely. Flex the PC muscle and hold to a count of nine. (Or some men find that flexing nine times in rapid succession works better. Try it both ways.) Resume thrusting with shallow strokes.

Alternate the Stimuli

When you are highly aroused, stop thrusting and make love to your partner manually or orally. Focus on giving her pleasure. By alternating intercourse with other forms of lovemaking, most men can make the encounter last longer. In sex therapy, this is sometimes referred to as the "stop/start technique."

Count the Strokes

Based on Taoist principles, which are all about holding back ejaculation, this one is simple, but men tell me it works. Count out sets of shallow, then deep, strokes. In the classic "set of nines," a man makes nine shallow strokes (without ever withdrawing completely), then one deep one, then eight shallow strokes, then two deep ones, and so forth.

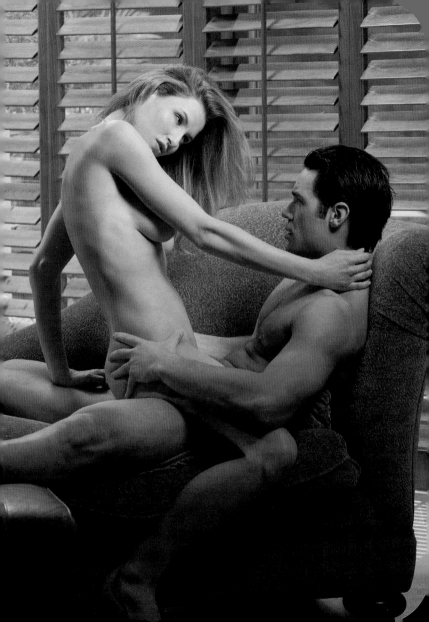

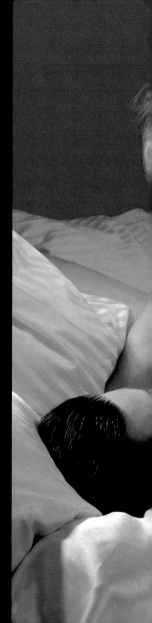

GAME 26

Pick a Card,
Any Card

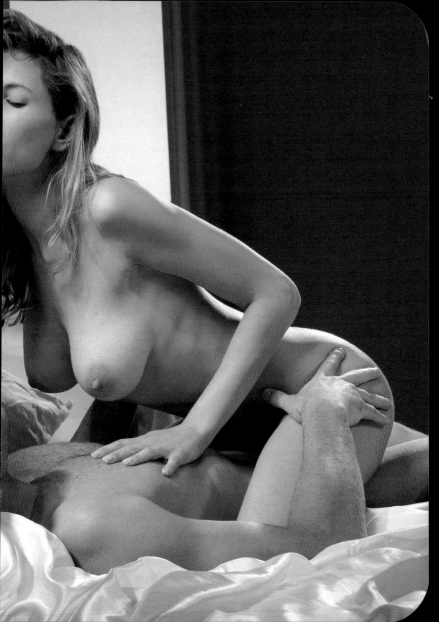

Pick a Card, Any Card

The Sexy Setup

Tell your lover you've got a game of cards that's sure to leave her satisfied. The premise is simple: Designate a playing card for each type of female orgasm, then let her pick one for your sex play. If she's been really good let her pick two or three cards!

Rules & Tools

If you're really creative you can make your own cards, but it's faster and easier to use a deck of playing cards and designate one card for each type of orgasm. You'll need between three and six cards, depending on what game you're playing; consider using the aces and queens, for example, or the ace, two, and three of a certain suit. Create a "cheat sheet" to remember that the ace of hearts represents a clitoral orgasm, the ace of diamonds a vaginal orgasm, the ace of spades a G-spot orgasm, and so on.

Playing the Game

Sweet and safe: Set up a romantic or sensual space for your sex play, whether that's in your bedroom or on a soft rug. This version of the game uses the three cards to represent the "tamest" types of orgasm: clitoral, vaginal, and G-spot. Have your lover pick a card, then focus on giving her that type of orgasm. Alternatively, let her have all three cards, but give her the choice of what order she wants her orgasms in. Feeling extra randy? Give her multiple versions of the same card. If you really want to draw out the pleasure, let her pick one card for the entire weekend!

Hot and spicy: This version of the game is a little more adventurous! Designate three additional cards to represent an anal orgasm, an extra-genital orgasm, and a blended orgasm (see Chapter 6). If she picks the anal card, plan on spending a lot of time licking her anus and/or inserting your well-lubed fingers and gently massaging. Working on an extra-genital orgasm? She's more likely to have this type after she's experienced a clitoral orgasm, so throw in a freebee and then turn all your attention to fondling, sucking, licking, pinching, or massaging her nipples, breasts, inner thighs, lower back, or other very sensitive areas. If she picks the blended orgasm card, ask which combination she prefers: Clitoris and vagina together? Clitoris and anal play? G-spot inter-course and anal play? Any way you cut it, she's sure to hit the jackpot!

Connect the Dots

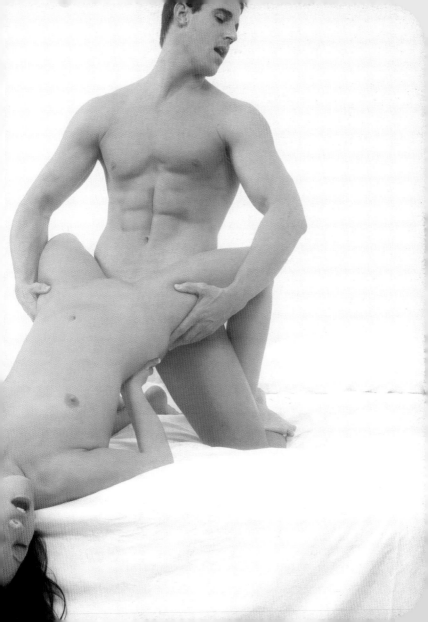

Connect the Dots

The Sexy Setup

No surprise here: You can heighten your sex play and orgasms by hitting each other's hot spots during oral and manual stimulation. Why not play a game of mutual hot spot exploration?

Rules & Tools

The sky's the limit with this game—bring along your vibrator, a cock ring for him, or some silk ties for light bondage.

Playing the Game

Hot and spicy (for her): During manual foreplay, stroke her AFE zone, then the G-spot, and back again. Use clockwise strokes followed by counterclockwise strokes. (Reminder: The AFE zone is a small, sensitive patch of textured skin at the top of the vagina close to the cervix. Stroking the AFE zone makes almost any woman lubricate immediately. The G-spot is that spongy mass of rough tissue located on the front wall of the vagina about halfway between the pubic bone and the cervix.) If you're going down on her, don't overlook her U-spot, or the tiny area of tissue above the opening of the urethra (and right below the clitoris). Shift from the C-spot to the U-spot when she is close to orgasm. Tease her by going back and forth until she can't take it anymore.

Hot and spicy (for him): Don't feel badly if you can't deep throat his penis without gagging. Concentrate your attention during fellatio on the H-spot (the head of the penis) and the R area (the visible line along the center of the scrotum); alternatively, stroke his P zone (the 1-inch area between the anus and the base of the scrotum). Connect these three dots and chances are he won't notice *or* care that you don't take the entire shaft into your mouth!

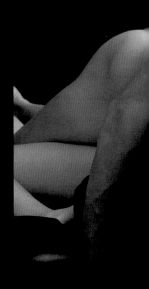

Hot Spot
Intercourse

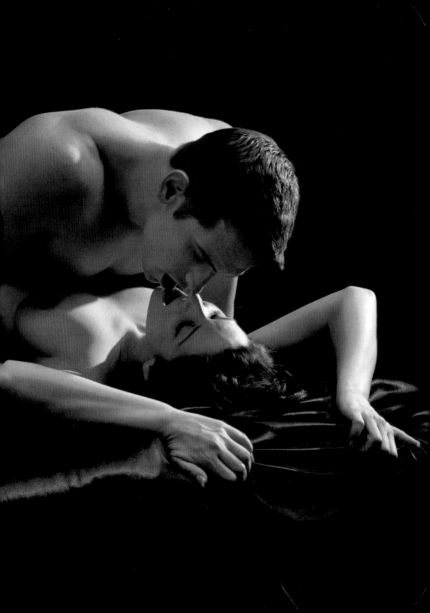

Hot Spot Intercourse

The Sexy Setup

Here's a fun game that combines hitting the hot spots and intercourse—what more could you ask for? Tell your lover you've got a game that's sure to hit all the right spots—and send him over the edge!

Rules & Tools

Be forewarned: Some of these positions may take a little practice, and some require a certain amount of flexibility! Set a sexy scene, dim the lights, and do some light stretches beforehand to get warmed up and build the sexual tension.

Playing the Game

Sweet and safe: In the missionary position, put your feet on his shoulders or pull your knees up to your chest and place your feet flat against his chest. Alternatively, have him hold your legs with his forearms under the knees. If you're on top, either lean back or forward, which is more effective at hitting the hot spots than riding straight up and down.

When using the spoon position, lie on your side with your back to him, bent slightly at the knees and waist. He enters you from behind, also bent slightly at the knees and waist.

Hot and spicy: Try the X position, which is adapted from the *Kama Sutra* position called "Woman acting the part of man." Imagine that your bodies form an X, with the connection at the genitals. He sits at the edge of the bed with his back straight and one leg outstretched on the bed, the other outstretched toward the floor, or, if he prefers, braced up on a straight-backed chair placed by the bed. Support your back with pillows, then sit astride your partner with both legs braced on his shoulders.

Drawwwww Out His Pleasure

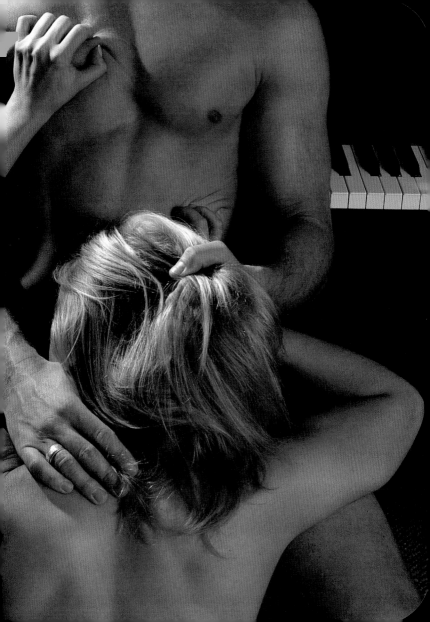

Drawwwww Out His Pleasure

The Sexy Setup

Text your lover and tell him you've got a game to play that's designed especially for him. The goal: to prolong his pleasurable sensations as long as possible without launching the rocket!

Rules & Tools

Set a sexy scene, whether that means making the bed with silk sheets or setting up a love nest in front of a burning fireplace. Dim the lights or light some candles, open a bottle of wine, and stash some lubricant or sex toys nearby for use if desired.

Playing the Game

Sweet and safe: First things first: Heat up your man in whatever way you like best—kiss him all over, manhandle his penis, or perform oral sex—whatever it takes to get him hard and ready. Then practice the Three-Finger Draw, a simple and effective technique that's been used in China for five thousand years. As you're sucking his penis, locate the midpoint of his perineum, or that sensitive area between the base of the testicles and the anus. As soon as you feel like he's going to come, curve the three longest fingers of your right hand very slightly and apply pressure—not too light and not too hard—to this spot. The trick is in finding the right spot and applying the pressure in the nick of time, which may take a little practice. Chances are he won't complain if you need to try, try again!

Hot and spicy: This technique, called the Big Draw, requires your lover to have a strong PC muscle (see 59). Heat him up as only you know best, then outline the technique. When he feels he's just about to come, have him stop thrusting and pull back to approximately 1 inch of penetration (but don't withdraw completely). Have him flex the PC muscle and hold to a count of nine, or flex nine times in rapid succession. (Have him try it both ways!) Resume thrusting with shallow strokes and repeat! Ready to step it up? Have him practice a Taoist technique called Count the Strokes. As he's thrusting, have him count out sets of shallow, then deep, strokes. In the classic "set of nines," he makes nine shallow strokes (without ever withdrawing completely), then one deep one, then eight shallow strokes, then two deep ones, and so forth. If you lose yourself in this game, whose counting, anyway?

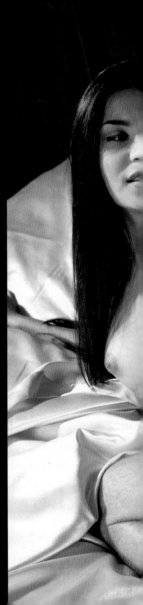

Spike My Oh!

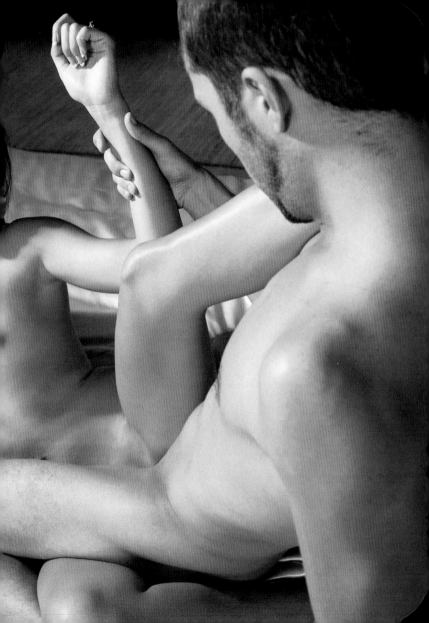

Spike My Oh!

The Sexy Setup

Every man does something special just before he's
going to orgasm. The goal of this game? To identify his
"moment" and spike his orgasm, otherwise known as
triggering it yourself!

Rules & Tools

You've got to do your homework before you can play this
game: Pay attention to the subtle signs that your lover is
close to coming, whether he holds his breath, breathes
more intensely, or makes a certain sound. Once you've
studied (and verified!) his particular moment, pull the
shades, light some candles, and wear your sexiest lingerie.

Playing the Game

Sweet and safe: Use your favorite moves to get your man
fully aroused. When you feel he's ready to come, spike his
orgasm, or "trigger" it yourself, by pinching, or biting
his nipples right at the moment of orgasm. Another easy
but effective maneuver: pause. If he's on top, grab his
buttocks at the moment of orgasm. Use your PC muscle
to pull him in a little deeper, and make eye contact with

him. Ready to step it up? Just as he's about to come, stimulate his G-spot with your thumb or finger pressed gently on his perineum. Alternatively, if he's comfortable, insert a well-lubed finger inside his anus to stimulate the G-spot from inside.

Hot and spicy: If he's on top and close to orgasm, grab his hip bones or buttocks and rock him, side to side, or back and forth. When you control the direction of his pelvic moments, you also control the speed of thrusting and the depth of penetration. To him, it feels like you are pulling the orgasm out of him in a very explosive way. Alternatively, if you're on top and he's close to orgasm, put your hands on his hips and pull him toward you. Keep your body weight on your knees so you don't bear down on his hips. Want to give him something really special? Fellate him to orgasm. When you feel he's ready to come, take his pelvis in both hands and rock him toward you so that he goes deeper into your mouth. Ready for the ultimate move? Master the Butterfly Quiver. When he's very hard, move so you're on top. Flex your PC muscle in a continuous pattern of tightening (as you pull him inside) and releasing (as you push him out), replicating the pattern of a butterfly's pulsating wings.

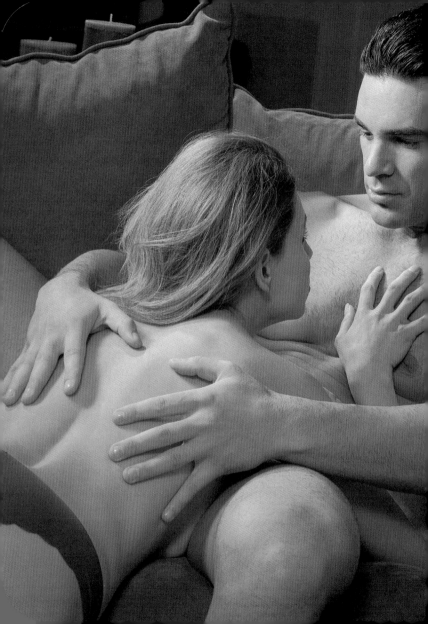

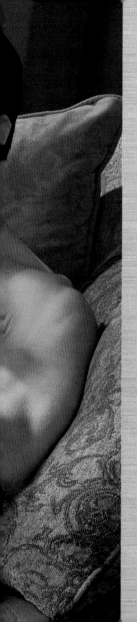

Eat Me Right and On Your Knees: Spectacular Oral Sex Techniques

For women, oral sex can serve as both foreplay and sex unto itself; for men, bringing your lover to orgasm via cunnilingus before intercourse ensures everyone gets the big Oh!

Eat Me Right

Here's a step-by-step process for perfecting
oral sex, or cunninlingus, on your female lover.

Step #1: After you have kissed, stroked, and fondled
the rest of her body so she is very aroused, get into a
position comfortable for both of you. She can lean against
pillows, either with her legs open, knees bent, and feet flat,
or with her legs outstretched and open, forming a V. You
can lie or kneel between her legs, or come in from the side
and wrap her leg around your shoulders. Or she
can straddle your face and lower her clitoris
to your mouth.

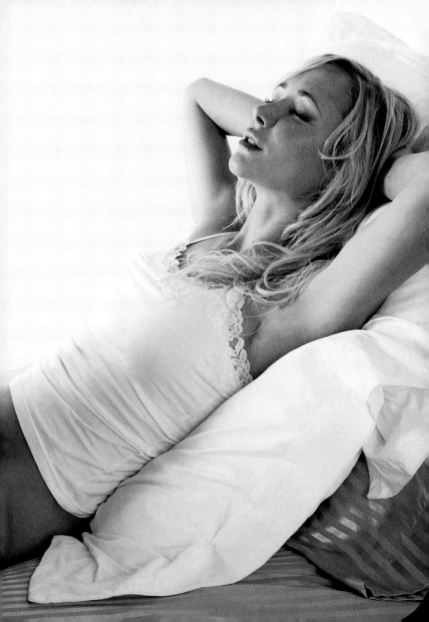

Step #2: Gently part her labia. Holding her lips open, lift the clitoral hood. If her clitoris is well back inside the hood—an "innie"—gently run your fingers along the side of the hood to expose the clitoris. (You may have to keep one hand in this position.)

Step #3: Lick the delicate tissue along the sides and above and below her clitoris with long, broad, *gentle* strokes of the tongue.

Step #4: Experiment with your tongue strokes, paying close attention to her responses. She will let you know how much pressure she wants, but if she doesn't, ask her if this feels good or what she likes best.

Step #5: Put your lips around the sides of her clitoris. Hold them in a pursed position as you gently suck. Alternate the sucking with licking of the surrounding tissues.

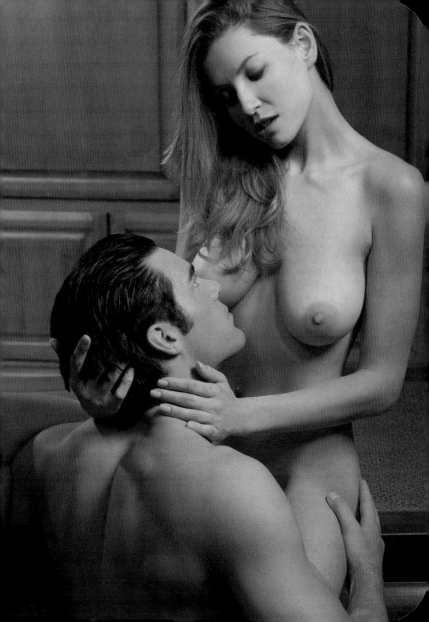

Step #6: If she likes direct stimulation of the clitoris—some women do, some don't—lick and suck it.

Step #7: Cover the clitoral shaft area with your mouth. Suck gently around the sides of her clitoris. Stimulate her labia with your hand or stroke her inner thighs, tease her nipples, or alternate manual stimulation. Don't move your mouth from her clitoris now if she wants to reach orgasm.

The Cunnilingus Power Move

If she's shy about cunnilingus, she may need to feel she's the one in control, not you. Giving her the power allows her to surrender on her own terms. Become her supplicant.

Kneel before her as she sits in a chair or on the side of the bed. Knead her buttocks softly as you bury your face in her vulva. Inhale deeply, and sigh happily. You are her willing oral servant now.

Begin licking from her knees up to her inner thighs. Manually stimulate her labia, vulva, vagina, and finally her clitoris while you give her thighs little sucking kisses. By the time your mouth surrounds her clitoris, she will have melted into you, inhibitions shed.

Giving a Great Blow Job

Here's a step-by-step technique for giving the perfect blow job—my technique, The Basic Black Dress of Blow Jobs. If you really want to cement the bond between you and your lover, swallow his semen when he comes!

Step #1: Kiss and lick his inner thighs while pulling down ever so slightly on his scrotum. With your finger pads, gently touch or scratch his testicles. Put his balls carefully into your mouth one at a time (assuming he likes this) and roll them around. Then, again, ever so gently, pull them down with your mouth.

Step #2: While you're attending to his balls, run you fingers lovingly up and down the shaft of his penis.

Step #3: Get into a comfortable position, kneeling at his side on the bed, at a right angle to his body, or kneeling between his legs. Or you can bring him down to the edge of the bed and kneel on the floor. Wet your lips and make sure that they cover your teeth. Run your tongue around the head of his penis to moisten it.

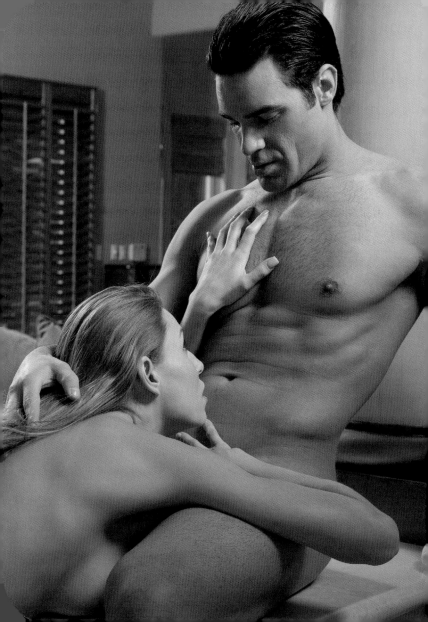

Step #4: Hold the base of his penis firmly in one hand. With the other hand, you can form a circle with your thumb and forefinger—what sex experts call the "ring and the seal"—to elongate your mouth and prevent him from going in farther than you would like. Use that hand in a twisting motion as you fellate him. Or, if his erection is not firm, you can use both hands (wrapped around the shaft) in an upward twisting stroke.

Step #5: Circle the head with your tongue in a swirling motion, and then work your tongue in long strokes up and down his shaft. Now, back to the head.

Step #6: Follow the ridge of the corona with your tongue while working the shaft with your hands, the penis sandwiched between them.

Step #7: Strum the frenulum with your tongue. Lick the raphe.

Step #8: Make eye contact with him from time to time.

Step #9: Do at least 10 to 20 seconds of this showy move: Repeatedly pull his penis into your mouth, then push it out, using suction while keeping the tongue in motion.

Step #10: Go back to the head. Swirl your tongue around it. Suck the head. Swirl. Suck. Repeat. Repeat.

Step #11: Follow his lead if he pulls back from stimulation. He's telling you that he's going to reach orgasm if you don't stop.

Swallowing

If you don't stop, you have two options: Swallow or let his semen dribble out of your mouth. Swallowing is not really difficult—and he will love you for it. A man feels totally accepted and loved by a woman who swallows his semen.

Position yourself so that his ejaculate will shoot straight down your throat. An easy way of doing this is to lie on your back with your head off the bed. Your mouth and throat will form a smooth line. Have him straddle your face for the elegant finish to the perfect blow job.

Does Size Make a Difference?

Oh, yes, it does to many women. This is one place where even women who prefer a large penis can see some advantage in a small one. You can easily deep throat the small penis. Your gag reflex is less likely to kick in. And who doesn't feel like an oral genius when she pulls that off?

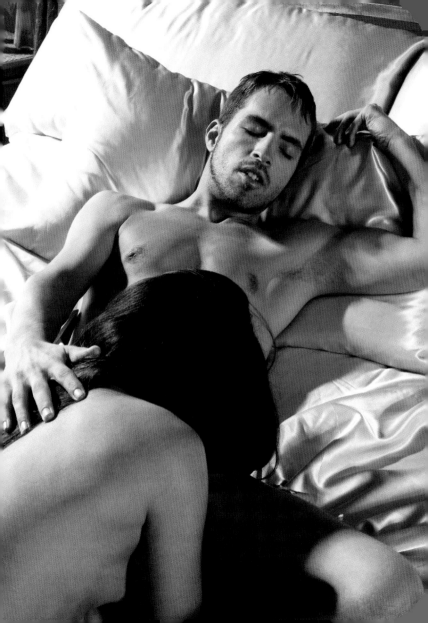

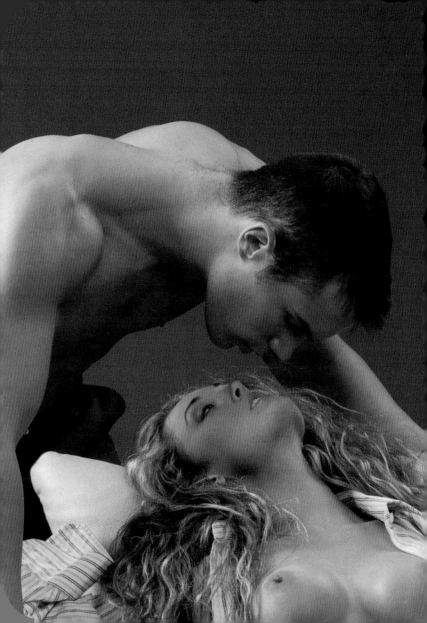

If your lover is well endowed, however, just concentrate on the top third of his penis. Supplement that with manual attention to the rest of the shaft, his testicles, and his perineum. Occasionally, adjust your position to allow you to take in all or most of his length. Here are a few ways to do this:

1. Kneel in front of him, bringing your mouth straight over the head of his penis. Now lower your head.

2. Have him lie on his side. Now you lie beside him with your head at penis level and take him into your mouth. The sideways angle gives you more control because he doesn't thrust as vigorously into your mouth as he does when he's flat on his back.

3. Lie on your back with your head over the edge of the bed. Have him kneel over you and thrust gently into your mouth. Control the depth of penetration with the ring and the seal.

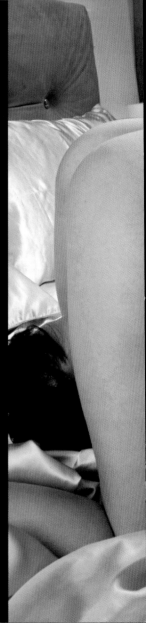

Classic 69
(and Then Some!)

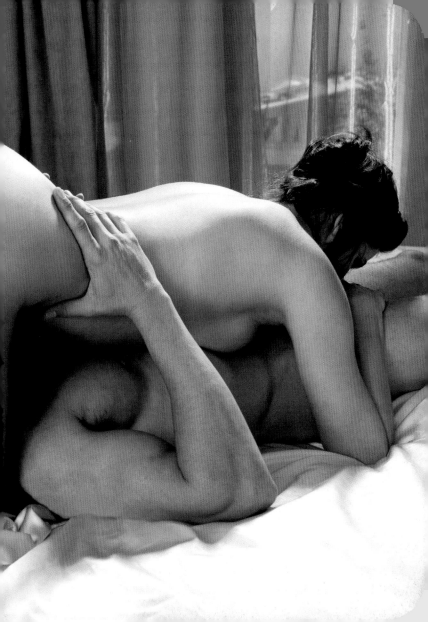

Classic 69 (and Then Some!)

The Sexy Setup

This is an easy game to pitch to your lover: You'll both get your share of oral pleasure. What's more, while everyone knows the meaning of 69, you may learn a few new variations on this classic position for oral sex!

Rules & Tools

This game takes a little concentration, as you're going to lick, suck, and use your tongue to give him (or her) a mind-blowing orgasm while he (or she) returns the favor. This may take practice, so don't beat yourself up if you lose yourself in your orgasm and have to pick up the reins and finish his afterward.

Playing the Game

Sweet and safe: Lie side by side with your lover, and rest your head on her inner thigh. (She can rest her head on your inner thigh.) Imagine her genital area as a flower that you are slowly and gently going to open up using your tongue and lips. Gently tease and kiss around her outer labia, using your fingers to part them slightly.

Use your tongue to feel for her inner lips, then flick her clitoris once or twice. Insert a finger into her vagina or her anus, then slowly increase the intensity and duration of your tongue on her clitoris. Use your fingers to gently expose the clit completely and use gentle laps of your tongue to bring her over the top. As you do this, ask your lover to practice her favorite oral sex techniques on your rock-hard penis.

Hot and spicy: Try these variations on the classic 69: Have your lover lie on top of you, facing your feet, knees at your shoulders and her genitals in your face. Prop a pillow under your head so you can reach her clitoris without straining your neck! Alternatively, lie on top of her and bury your head between her thighs. Your penis will dangle right over her mouth! Last but not least, try the Curled 69: Curl into a tucked position for a tighter, more intimate version of the classic oral sex thriller.

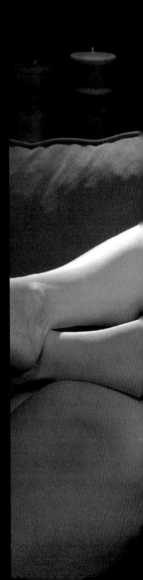

GAME 32

Queen for a Day

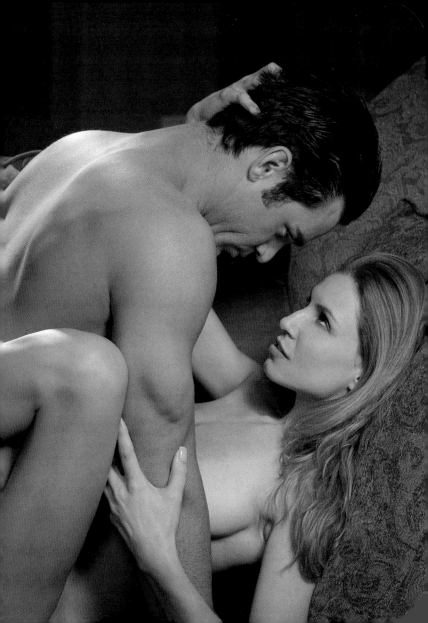

Queen for a Day

The Sexy Setup

Tell your lover you're her adoring knight, and you want to treat her like a queen. Specifically, you've got a seat of honor that promises hours of pleasure!

Rules & Tools

This is all about pleasuring your lover, so be prepared to spend some time on your knees, exploring all her most glorious treasures. If you want to get into role-playing, dress like a squire or knight, and ask her to dress like a queen. Then set up a throne by draping furs or velvet over a chair and giving her a crown. Bring along a silk tie for blindfolding.

If you're not on a bed or other soft surface, put a blanket or pillow under her knees. Explain to her that she's in control—while you're there to pleasure her orally, she can control the intensity by moving up and down on your tongue. If she needs something to hold on to, position yourselves so she can lean her hands against the wall.

Playing the Game

Sweet and safe: Lead your lover to her throne, perhaps blindfolded so she doesn't know what awaits her. Slowly and seductively remove her clothing, or, if you're playing a game of stolen royal love along the lines of Catherine Howard, the wife of Henry VIII who had an affair with Thomas Culpeper, lift up her skirts and bury your face in her vulva. Start by kissing her inner thighs and taking in the smell and taste of her vulva. Give her genitals long, slow, wet kisses, then introduce your tongue for exploring her labia, crevices, and clitoris. Find a rhythm she likes to give her a mind-blowing orgasm fit for a queen! Alternatively, have your lover kneel above your face so you can use your kisses and tongue to explore her labia and clitoris; run your tongue from her vagina to her anus and back again, all the while gently massing her buttocks. Put a finger or two inside her vagina and play with her G-spot while you bring her to orgasm with your tongue.

(continued on page 258)

Hot and spicy: In this scenario, pretend you are a foreign knight who has taken the queen hostage. Your duty: not to hurt her, but to pleasure her beyond her wildest dreams. Lead her to her throne, but then tie her hands to the chair. Spread her legs and tie her legs to the chair as well. Now she's your captive, and you can tease her until she screams for mercy—or moans with pleasure! Ready to step it up? Put together a "Royal Tool Kit" full of her favorite sex toys and props, then use them one by one while she's strapped to the chair. Use a finger vibrator to stimulate her nipples while you lick her clitoris, or bring her to orgasm manually while you penetrate her with a dildo. Talk about your majesty's secret service!

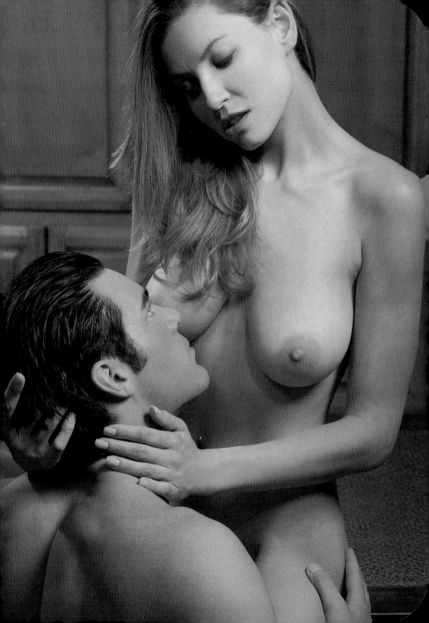

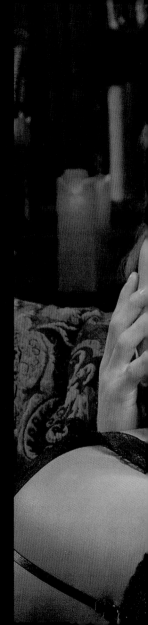

GAME 33

Oral Sex Slave

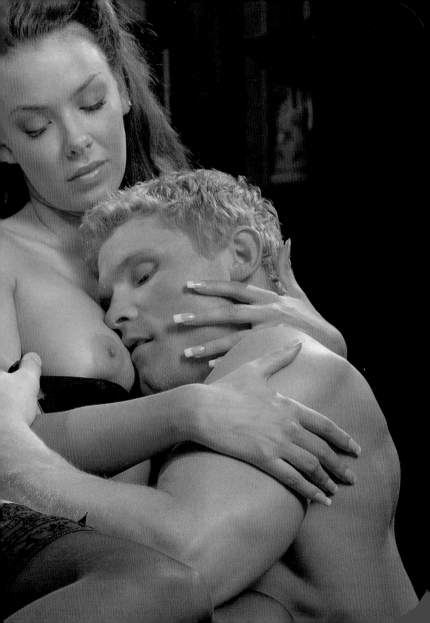

Oral Sex Slave

The Sexy Setup

What man doesn't relish the thought of his own personal sex slave? But the twist in this game is that it's all about pleasuring him using oral sex. Ladies, get on your knees and service your master!

Rules & Tools

Set up a pleasure den using soft blankets, furs, or silk sheets. Dress the part as you see fit: Wear your sexiest lingerie and high heels, a maiden's dress with no undergarments, a leather jacket and boots (otherwise naked!), or a collar and nothing else. Bring along soft ties for gentle bondage if desired.

Playing the Game

Sweet and safe: Lead your lover to his pleasure den, and ask him where he most likes to be kissed. Start kissing him there, but then take your kisses to his neck, his chest, his belly, and downward. Kiss him all over, but avoid the genitals and tease him until he orders you to touch him *there*. Then suck, nibble, and bite your way around until he orders you to make him come. Alternatively, lie down and have him kneel in front of you so his penis is right in front of your mouth (you may need a pillow or two to get the angle right). Hold his penis with one hand and explore his backside with the other; fondle his testicles, insert a finger in his anus, or just lightly trace your fingertips along his perineum as you suck him off.

Hot and spicy: Before you begin the actual sex play, ask him what he'd like to eat and drink, then sit on his lap and hand feed him grapes or let him sip champagne. Shower him with affection while he relaxes and unwinds, but then surprise him suddenly by tying him to the chair (a short struggle will turn you both on!) and removing just enough of his clothes to reveal his genitals. Although he's the master, he's also your prisoner, and you intend to draw out your pleasurable torture. Undress seductively and tease him in a sexy manner, all the while knowing he cannot touch you. When he's sufficiently turned on, get on your knees and suck him off as you know best.

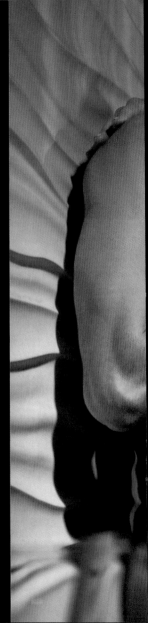

GAME 34

8 Days a Week

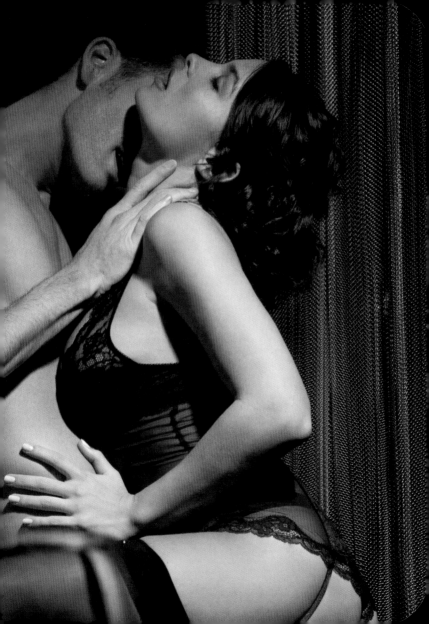

8 Days a Week

The Sexy Setup

Remember the Beatles song, "8 Days a Week"? This extended game is all about drawing out the pleasure—and teasing your lover over several days—in order to give him the orgasm of his life.

Rules & Tools

This game doesn't have to be played over 7 days. It could take place over a weekend, with the pleasure given every few hours—or you can really make the work week hum by by giving a small amount of pleasure every night, but holding off on letting him come until the last night. The rules are simple: Use your oral sex techniques every day (or every few hours) to stimulate him, but don't let him come until you're ready. It will be a challenge for you to pull away, but even harder for him to know he's got to wait for his orgasm!

Playing the Game

Sweet and safe: Sing to the tune of the Beatles song, but use these naughty lyrics instead:

Ooh I need your cock, babe,
Guess you know it's true.
Hope you need my lips, babe,
Just like I need you.
Hold me, kiss me, hold me, suck you.
I ain't got nothin' but blow jobs,
Eight days a week.

Day #1: Wet your lips and run your tongue around the head of his penis to moisten it. Hold the base of his penis firmly in one hand, then form the ring and the seal with your other hand. Use that hand in a twisting motion as you fellate him. Get him stimulated, but stop well before orgasm.

Day #2: Circle the head of his penis with your tongue in a swirling motion, and then work your tongue in long strokes up and down his shaft. Again, get him stimulated but don't let him come.

Day #3: Follow the ridge of the corona with your tongue while working the shaft with your hands, the penis sandwiched between them.

Day #4: Strum the frenulum with your tongue and lick the raphe. Make eye contact with him from time to time.

(continued on page 268)

Day #5: Repeatedly pull his penis into your mouth, then push it out, using suction while keeping the tongue in motion.

Day #6: Go back to the head. Swirl your tongue around it. Suck the head. Swirl. Suck. Repeat. Repeat.

Day #7: Use one or all of the above techniques to get him off!

Hot and spicy: Use the timeline and techniques already listed, but step it up by introducing gentle bondage, an anal butt plug, or gentle nipple clamps. Ready for even racier sex play? Bring a friend along, blindfold your lover, and take turns stimulating him. Remember, don't let him come until the final day!

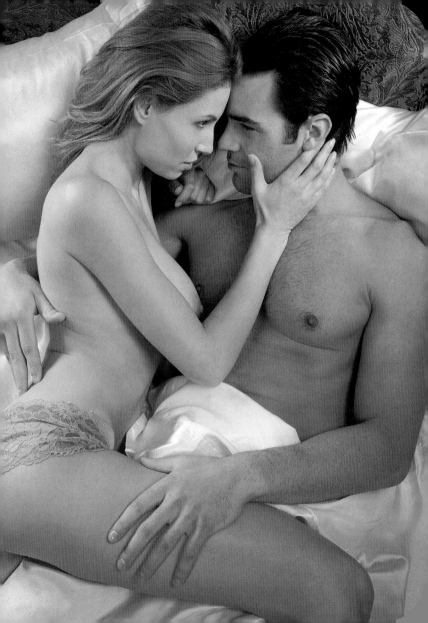

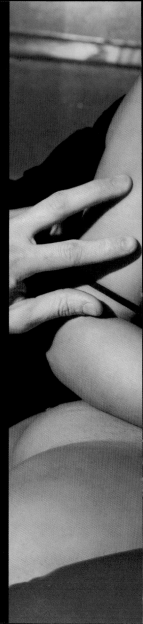

tranger Danger

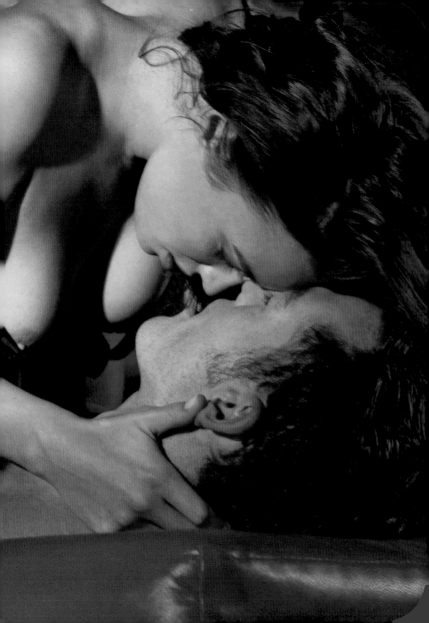

Stranger Danger

The Sexy Setup

This is a great game to play with a longtime lover, as it brings out the "danger" and "secret" elements of having sex with a stranger or in a public place. Tell your lover you're going to play a game where he's the pickup target, but you're calling the shots.

Rules & Tools

Make a plan ahead of time with your lover, then send him a sexy note to remind him of the details. "Meet me at Oliver's at 8 pm; be sure to bring a hard-on."

Playing the Game

Sweet and safe: Dress as if you're out to pick up a man: Try a new top with a plunging neckline that he hasn't seen or a short skirt that shows your legs. Instruct your lover to find a spot at the bar, order a drink, and relax. Then do your best to flirt him up: Play hard to get, act like a tease, or flirt openly. Draw out the pickup as long as possible to heighten the tension, then lead him to your car and continue teasing him by licking and sucking on his penis. If you want to draw out the pleasure, leave him panting for more but go back to the bar. You can always pick up where you left off once you get home!

Hot and spicy: Play the part of a slut or prostitute. Tease him with your eyes or hands, brush up against him suggestively, or touch his package when no one's looking. Whisper what you'd like to do to him while you lean over and expose your cleavage. Alternatively, invite a female friend to join in (but don't tell your lover). Ask your friend to flirt with your man openly—a little competition can add some spice to the situation. Have a secret word for when it's time for her to head home. Once he's hot and hard, take him by the hand and give him a steamy blow job in the men's bathroom or a hidden closet—the fear of getting caught will only intensify his orgasm!

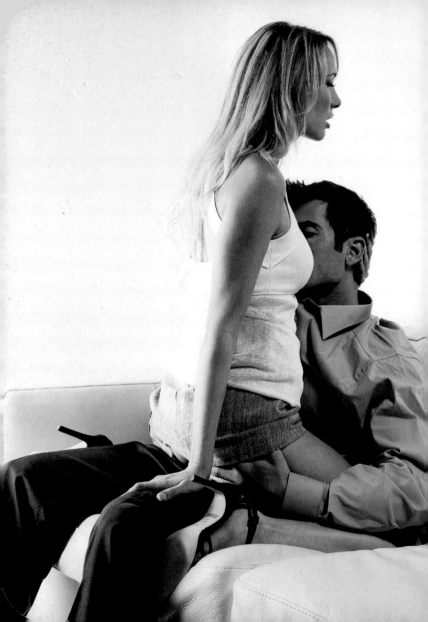

CHAPTER 8

Beyond the Obvious (Quickies and Anal Orgasms)

This is the place to let go of some of your assumptions about orgasm. Do you think quickies are something women do for men—because she won't come but he will? Do you believe that anal orgasms are myths— maybe myths perpetrated by husbands who want anal sex? These things—and more—are possible!

How to Make a Quickie Work for Her, Too

There isn't always time for the kind of extended foreplay and long lovemaking sessions that favor women's orgasms. Modern couples, especially two-careers-plus-kids couples, don't have that kind of time every day, even most days. They put sex off 'til Saturday night. Maybe they even avoid touching one another in bed because they don't want to start something that one or both has neither the time nor the energy to finish. The weekend comes and someone has a cold, the in-laws are visiting, social obligations have piled up. Soon sex avoidance becomes a habit. Before they know what has happened to them, they become that couple that can't remember the last time they had sex.

Unless you have the luxury of time every day of the week, you need to learn the art of the quickie. Sex begets sex. The more you have, the more you want. The less you have—well, you don't want to go there, do you?

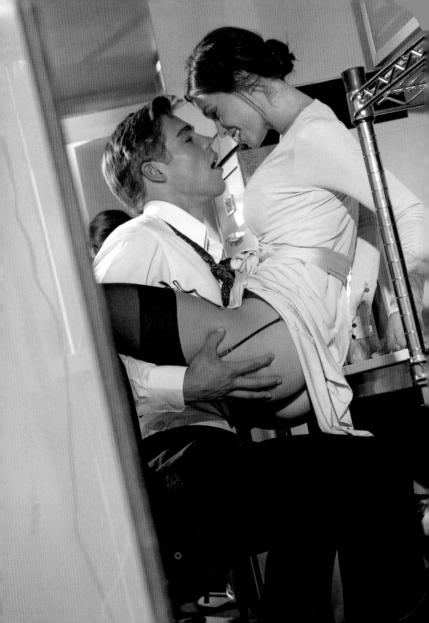

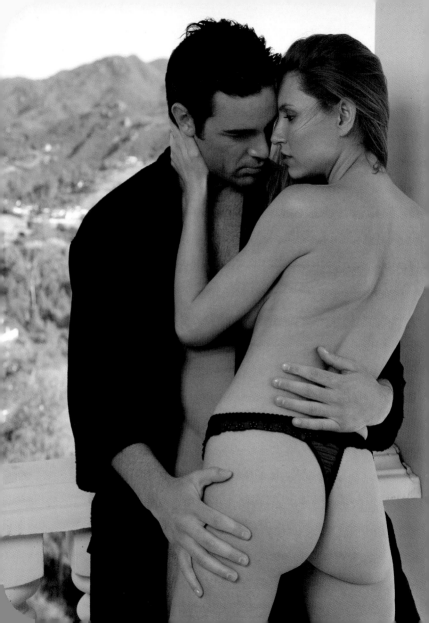

Myths and Misconceptions of Quickies

Keep the following myths in mind; remember, these are *not* true:

- Women can't come during a quickie.

- If you let a man "have" a quickie, he won't want to do it any other way.

- Only couples who are new to each other have the kind of passionate desire that fuels a quickie.

- It's over before she's had a chance to lubricate.

- A quickie is just another name for "premature ejaculation sex."

The Quickie Essentials

Want a quickie to work for both of you? Here are some tips:

- **Sex your brain:** Sure, it's possible that lust takes you by surprise. You get swept up in passion. You melt at the sight of him. You grow erect when she unbuttons her blouse. But if you can't wait for lust to take you like a pirate swooping up booty, then encourage your sexual thoughts and fantasies, especially just before you'll have time for a quickie. Put sex in your head.

- **Prepare your body:** Use a lube like Liquid Silk or KY vaginal moisturizer (in applicators like tampons) that she can put in a little ahead of time. She can use a Pocket Rocket vibe to rev up her clitoris. In less than two minutes, she'll be ready.

- **Redefine sex:** "Sex" doesn't have to mean intercourse. You can skip the foreplay this time. Really. If she's lubed and revved up and he has an erection, you're good to go. Plus intercourse that takes place in a secret place or unusual position adds a sense of urgency and excitement to the encounter!

- **Touch her clitoris:** Use your hand or a finger vibe, but don't neglect clitoral stimulation.

- **Be edgy:** There are so many places to have a quickie, especially since you don't take all your clothes off. The risk of being seen also adds an element of excitement.

Anal Sex Play

Anal? Really? Really. The anal orgasm is not just a theory promulgated by men trying to get women to try anal intercourse. The anus, in both sexes, is rich in nerve endings. Stimulating it does bring pleasure. Bring on the toys, fingers, and tongues, and see whether anal play arouses you before trying anal intercourse.

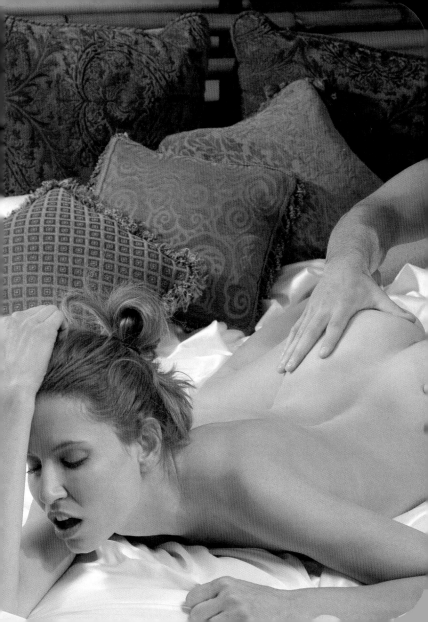

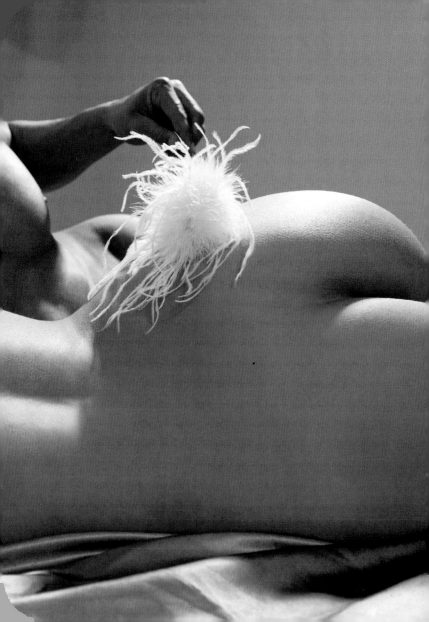

Anal Massage

1. Massage her buttocks using firm strokes. Then use light, teasing strokes—even gentle pinching—down the crack between her cheeks.
2. Separating the buttocks slightly, massage the innermost parts with somewhat gentler strokes than you used on the outer buttocks.
3. Apply the light, teasing strokes you used in her crack down to her anus. With a well-lubed finger, circle the anal opening lightly.
4. Using long strokes, begin massaging her buttocks again, starting at the base of the spine and continuing down the perineum.
5. Massage her perineum with your thumb or finger pad, exerting light pressure.
6. Put your finger in her anus and gently circle inside the opening. Now add a second finger. Rub them in and out in simulated intercourse.
7. Swap roles and do this to your man!

Anal Toys

Consider using the following anal toys:

- **Anal beads:** Made of jelly, plastic, or silicone, anal beads look like the necklaces made of pop beads that you had as a child. At the end of this string of beads is a large circular pull. You gently insert the (well-lubricated) beads, then pull them out, one bead at a time, for an *ooh-la-la* effect. Flexi Felix, made of silicone, is a high-quality product, with no rough edges on the beads, and it is easier to clean than the cheaper versions.

- **Butt plugs:** Varying in size and somewhat in shape, butt plugs are insertable wands that have a flared base so you don't have to worry about them getting lost up there. Used during masturbation, they will make you aware that your anal muscles really do clench in orgasm—and they will heighten that sensation. A preparation for anal sex, a butt plug opens the pathway. Some women find that using a butt plug during intercourse gives them a delicious feeling of double penetration. Use lots of lube. (And if he wants you to try a butt plug, why don't you ask him to try one, too?)

- **Anal vibrators or attachments:** Anal vibrators are specially designed for anal insertion. They are smaller—both shorter and thinner—than regular vibes.

Anal Intercourse

Before beginning, get the necessary props: a good lubricant, such as Astroglide (no scented oils, lotions, or petroleum jelly), and an anal condom, which is necessary to keep bacteria out of his urethra.

Step #1: Find the position. For men and women—especially beginners—the rear-entry position with your chest flat on the bed and your ass elevated is the easiest position.

Step #2: Lube up. Using strokes that you finds pleasurable, he generously lubes your anus and rectum.

Step #3: Start slowly. As he presses the head of his penis against your anus, relax the sphincter muscles in your rectum. Push the muscles out so that you are pushing onto him as he is pressing into you. He shouldn't force entry. Rather, you should bear down on the head of his penis until he is past the sphincter muscles.

Step #4: Begin thrusting. He begins to thrust slowly and carefully, following your lead. You control the depth and speed of penetration.

Step #5: Stimulate the clitoris. While he is thrusting, you (or he, but only if his fingers are clean) stimulate your clitoris.

Step #6: Stay clean (and safe). Afterward, don't let him insert his penis or fingers into your vagina until he has disposed of the condom and washed his hands. Remember, you both risk contracting a urinary tract infection from anal sex if the cleanliness rules are not followed scrupulously. No vaginal sex after anal sex until he has washed.

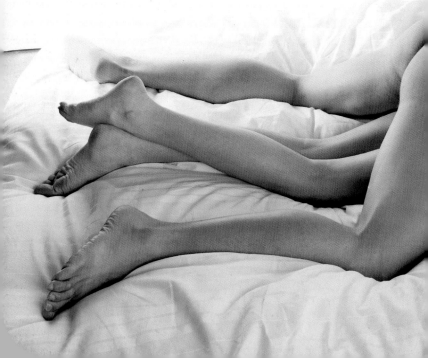

And keep this in mind: Porn films are vehicles for arousal, not how-to videos. So never mind that porn actors slide in and out of orifices with no time-outs for washing (and no specs of feces on their penises, either). That is not real life.

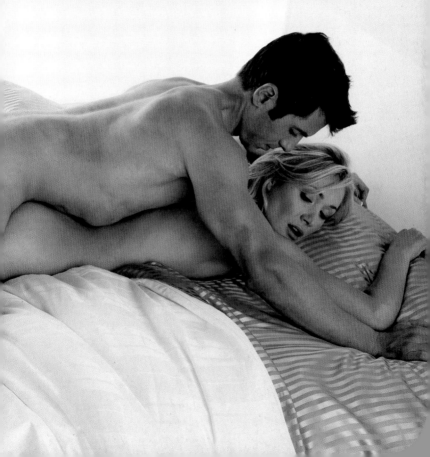

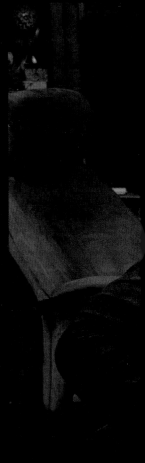
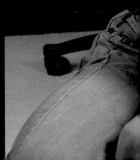

Dress for Quickie Success

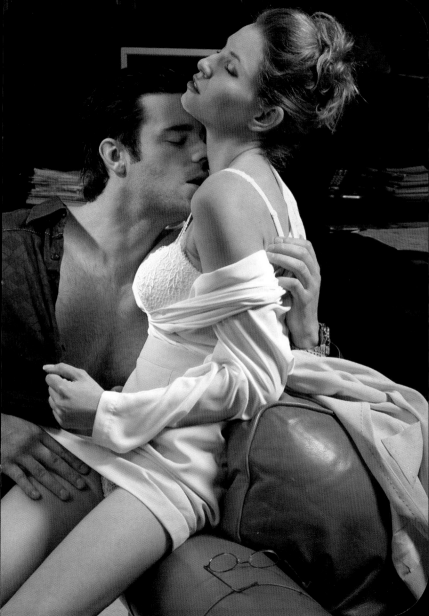

Dress for Quickie Success

The Sexy Setup

Here's a sexy "dress-up" game that's sure to get you both aroused—and give you ideas for how to dress for quickie success in the future!

Rules & Tools

Anything goes in this game, although the end goal is to walk away with several outfits or costumes that are perfect for quickie sex. Think of this as a road test for all your sexiest clothing that can be pushed aside, unzipped quickly, or just torn off! If you want, make a scorecard and rating system for your lover so he can rank your outfits. Remember, any score is a good score!

Playing the Game

Sweet and safe: If you're new to quickie sex, this is the perfect game for you. Set up a sexy "viewing" area for your lover, whether that's on your bed, in a relaxing chair, or lying naked on a rug! Dim the lights and fix him a cocktail, then ask him to play voyeur for a bit while you model some quickie outfits. Head into your closet and model a variety of push-aside costumes: Try a short skirt with no underwear, a zip-down sweater with no bra underneath, lingerie that can be easily pushed aside, and so on. Be sure to include one outfit that can be ripped off, such as an old t-shirt and a pair of his worn-out boxers. Have your lover rank each outfit for how much it turns him on and how easily he thinks it will work for quickie sex. Feeling randy? Move on to the hot and spicy version of this game.

Hot and spicy: Put each outfit to the test! Set up a timer and see how long it takes your lover to get to down to business, whether that means manhandling your breasts, fondling your buttocks, or exploring your clitoris with his tongue or fingers. If you're feeling especially sexy, try to fight him off—gentle horseplay can add to the excitement. And don't forget the outfit that can be ripped off—a little roughhousing can really heat up the action! Alternatively, set the timer and see how long it takes to reach orgasm using each different outfit.

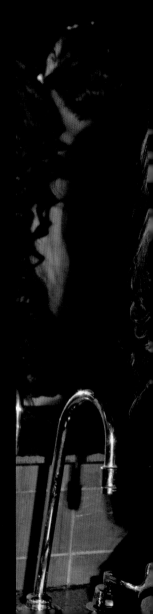

Quickie
Chinese Menu

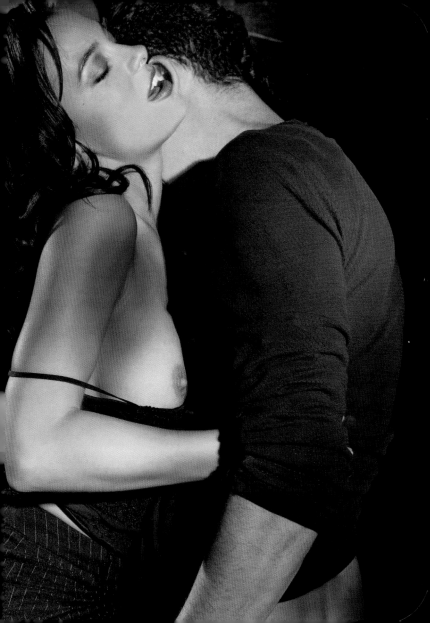

Quickie Chinese Menu

The Sexy Setup

You know the concept of a Chinese food menu—pick one dish from column A, another from column B, and so on until you've built your meal. This game works on the same premise, but you're picking what kind of quickie sex you want and where to have it. Tell your lover you've got a sexy menu of options that need testing, and he's an essential ingredient!

Rules & Tools

Set up a matrix together: Design a grid where column A represents all the different types of quickie sex and column B represents all the assorted places to have that sex. Use your imagination—pick a variety of places in your home, at your office, outdoors, or even in public places such as a furniture store or movie theater.

Playing the Game

Sweet and safe: Close your eyes and put your finger on one of the boxes in the matrix for a quickie surprise. Alternatively, work through the matrix together until there's a check in every box. Options include: Pretend you are meeting your lover in an empty conference room and time is of the essence. Do it in the backyard at midnight, in the restroom of your favorite pub, or in your mother's gazebo.

Hot and spicy: Add some of these locations to your matrix, then test them out one by one! Have mutual oral sex in the backseat of the car parked in the garage, while the kids are watching a video inside the house. Have sex in a standing position in your bedroom closet while your dinner guests are cleaning up the dishes. Visit your lover at his office and sit on his lap in a desk chair. Sit on top of the running dryer and have your man perform oral sex—the heat and vibrations of the dryer will add to the pleasure! Shopping at the mall? Suck off your man in the men's dressing room, or find a hidden room in a cavernous furniture store.

GAME 38

Anal Play 101

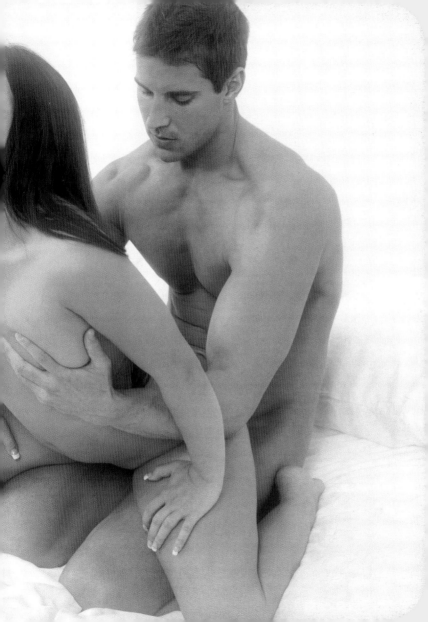

Anal Play 101

The Sexy Setup

If you've never experimented with anal sex play, here's the game for you. Tell your lover you're interested in exploring her back end, but promise to take it slow, talk it through, and change gears if anything feels awkward or uncomfortable. Then get ready to think about all things anal, all the time!

Rules & Tools

Set a sexy scene for your backdoor experimentation, and serve your lover a glass of wine or champagne if she's at all nervous about this idea. Bring along plenty of lubricant, use safe practices, and stash your favorite props (feathers or silk ties) and toys (butt plug, anal beads, or other toys) nearby if you sense she's at all comfortable with taking things a little further.

Playing the Game

Sweet and safe: Kiss her deeply and slowly undress her, taking time to caress her neck, arms, and breasts as you always do. Tell her how beautiful she is and how excited you are to experiment with new techniques together.

If she's really tense, consider bringing her to orgasm before you explore her backside, so she'll be more relaxed. Have her lie on her side or stomach, then gently massage her buttocks. Gently run a finger, feather, or a silk tie very lightly down her crack, then separate her buttocks as you go. Repeat this as necessary, making sure she's aroused before you move to the next step. Tease her buttocks apart using very light strokes, then circle closer to her anus, all the while kissing her lower back or the back of her neck. Apply lubrication to your finger and slowly tease the anal opening, then retreat. Repeat the tease-and-retreat technique until you're sure she's aroused, then gently insert your finger into her anus and circle inside the opening. Push and pull your finger in and out as if you were having sex; if she's interested, insert a second finger and continue the movement.

Hot and spicy: Try stimulating her clitoris with your other hand as you move your finger in and out of her anus. Alternatively, masturbate as you touch her anal area, then come onto her lower back. Ready for more advanced techniques? Use a set of anal beads on your lover: Lubricate the beads, insert them gently into her anus, then pull them out, one bead at a time, while you kiss her breasts or lick her clitoris. Use an anal plug while you have sex—your lover may find the double penetration expands her orgasm.

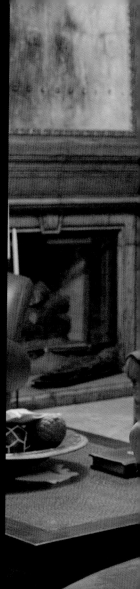

GAME 39

Beyond Doggie-Style

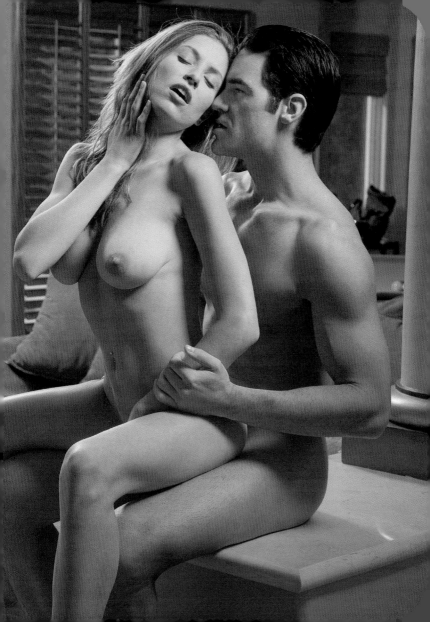

Beyond Doggie-Style

The Sexy Setup

If you've already had anal intercourse and you're ready for experimentation, this position game is just for you. Tell your lover you've got some new ideas for backdoor pleasure that are sure to get him off!

Rules & Tools

Have plenty of lubrication and be sure to use safe practices. Bring along your favorite vibrator if desired. Then let your imagination—or your flexibility—influence the direction of this game.

Playing the Game

Sweet and safe: If you're a beginner when it comes to anal sex, the doggie-style position is easiest. But if you're ready for some variation on that game, lie on your back with your legs straight up or your ankles resting on his shoulders. Have him kneel between your legs, lube things up, and thrust away! Alternatively, have him lie on his back, then lower yourself onto him, either facing him or facing away, or have him sit in a chair or on the bed, then lower yourself onto him, facing away. And the ultimate position for easy anal sex? Spoon style: Lie side by side, with your buttocks against his penis.

Hot and spicy: Try these more advanced moves for better anal sex. Stand together in a doorway, with you facing away from your lover. Let him penetrate you as you hold onto the doorframes for leverage! Lean over if you want it hard and deep. Alternatively, have him lie flat on his back, then lower yourself onto him but extend your body so you end up laying flat on top of him, your back to his chest. Ask him to kiss your neck and play with your clitoris as you have anal sex. Last but not least, have him sit on a chair, then lower yourself onto him. Bring along your vibrator and masturbate to clitoral orgasm while he enters your backdoor.

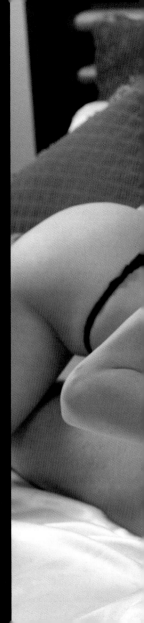

GAME 40

Backdoor Woman

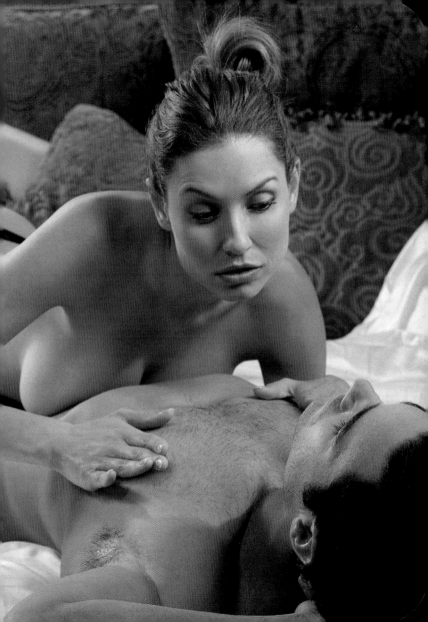

Backdoor Woman

The Sexy Setup

You've heard the phrase backdoor man? This time the roles are reversed: You get to control the action at your male lover's back door. Write your male lover a sexy note and tell him you want to explore his back door. Promise you'll be gentle and as you investigate his backside's assets, but you're sure there's some new pleasures zones worth exploring!

Rules & Tools

Line up a number of anal toys for this game and bring along plenty of lubrication. Have these (or other toys) on hand: butt plug, strap-on dildo, anal vibrator, anal beads, or any pocketsize or finger vibrator. Set up a low-lit, sexy scene for this game: Line a couch with fur, create a nest of soft blankets on the floor, or make your bed with silk sheets.

Playing the Game

Sweet and safe: If this is your lover's first time with anal play, take it slow. Dress in your sexiest lingerie and help him loosen up by serving him a drink. Then take out one of your toys and let him look at it close-up. Explain why you think it might turn him on, but be open if he's not interested and simply move on to the next toy. Kiss and caress him in your usual way, then slowly move to fondling and sucking his penis and nibbling his testicles. Try running a finger vibrator along his inner thighs, up to his testicles, and along his perineum. Be sure to ask if he likes the feeling, and if he does, continue with your back door play, perhaps inserting the butt plug or anal beads while you suck him off.

Hot and spicy: You know your man's open to any anal suggestion, so take it up a notch and explore your own fantasies. Lube up the strap on and give it to him up the ass like the strong and sexy backdoor woman you are, or just insert a vibrating butt plug and ride him like a cowgirl! Ready to step it up? Play a game of backdoor woman meets backdoor man. Both of you should chose your favorite butt plug, then have intercourse doggie style!

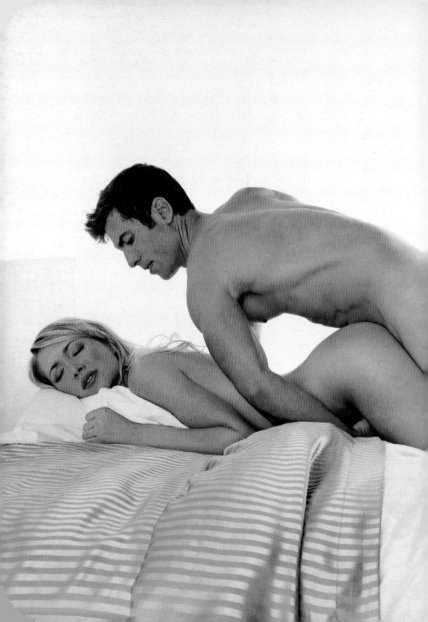

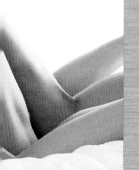

CHAPTER 9

Repeat After Me (Multiple Orgasms and Orgasm Positions)

Theoretically, every woman can have multiple orgasms because women do not have a refractory period. Only 10 percent of women report, having multiple orgasms, but striving to increase that percentage is a worthy goal!

Types of Multiples

There are four types of multiple orgasms:

- **Compounded single orgasms:** Each orgasm is distinct, separated by sufficient time so that prior arousal and tension have substantially resolved between orgasms.

- **Sequential multiples:** Orgasms are fairly close together—anywhere from two to ten minutes apart—with little interruption in sexual stimulation or level of arousal.

- **Serial multiples:** Orgasms are separated by seconds, or up to two or three minutes, with no or barely any interruption in stimulation or diminishment of arousal.

- **Blended multiples:** A mix of two or more of the above types. Very often women who are multiply orgasmic experience more than one type of multiple orgasm during a lovemaking session.

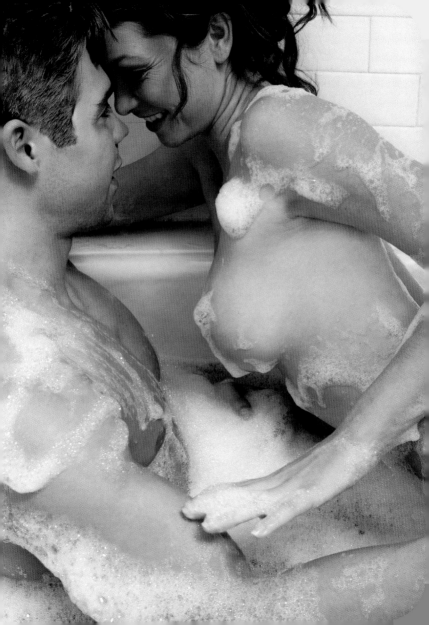

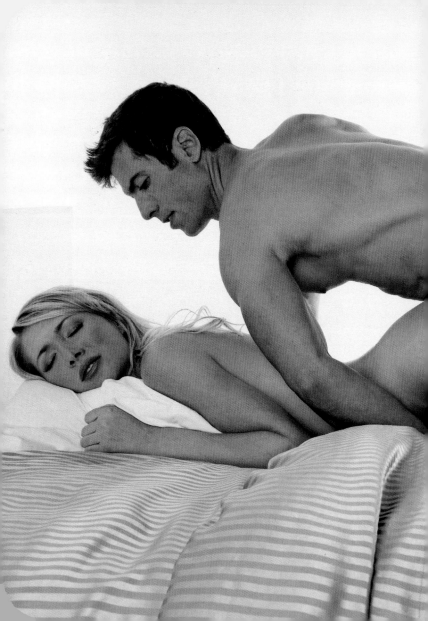

Encouraging Multiples

What can you do to encourage multiple orgasms?
Here are some tips:

- **Start warm:** Fantasize about the sexual encounter before it begins. Masturbate, but not to orgasm. Indulge in sensual cues, such as candles, music, perfume, and lingerie. Set time aside for longer-than-usual lovemaking.

- **Focus:** You must be focused solely on your pleasure to achieve multiples. If you are paying too much attention to him—even to pleasing him—you won't get there. You probably won't have them if you're tired, stressed, or angry, particularly with your lover. Mental attitude is crucial. Shut out intrusive thoughts and practice the principles of the Orgasm Loop.

- **Touch yourself:** A woman who has multiple orgasms is comfortable giving herself additional clitoral stimulation during sex.

What Can He Do to Help?

Unless you're masturbating to multiple orgasms, the pursuit is something of a joint effort. He won't mind at all. Men are somewhat in awe of the female ability to come and come again—and they feel like more powerful lovers if their woman does. Here are some ways he can help out:

- **Alternate stimuli:** During lovemaking, alternate physical stimuli. The first one or two orgasms, for example, may be via cunnilingus or manual stimulation. Rarely will a woman have multiples if you move from foreplay straight to intercourse.

- **Use your hands:** Touch her clitoris. When she isn't stroking her clitoris, you probably should be. Don't leave her clitoris alone for too long if you want to help her reach orgasm multiple times. If she is G-spot responsive, use your fingers to stimulate her G-spot while you perform cunnilingus.

- **Try the Flame:** For some women, this is the ultimate cunnilingus stroke. Pretend the tip of your tongue is a candle flame. In your mind's eye, see that flame flickering in the wind. Move your tongue rapidly around the sides of her clitoris, above and below it, as the candle flame moves.

Orgasm Positions

When a woman says, "I can't come with him," what she usually means: "I can't come with any man during intercourse alone." That's normal. Whether you reach orgasm

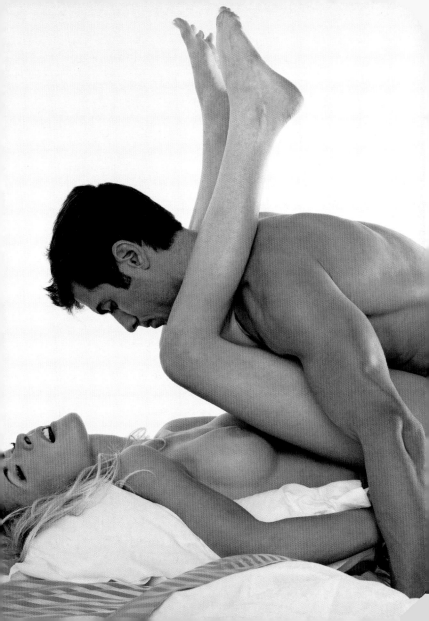

or you don't has little to do with him and much to do with you. Here's how to reach orgasm with your partner.

Manual Stimulation During Intercourse, in Any Position

One of you has to touch your clitoris and the surrounding tissue during intercourse, or you should bring a vibe to bed with you. One or the other needs only to insert a finger or two, or the flat or the side of a hand between your bodies, and stroke. If you're too shy to touch yourself in front of him or to tell him how you like to be touched, just take his hand, put it there, and move against it.

You can also use a finger vibe, wear a strap-on vibe, or masturbate to the point where orgasm is imminent before intercourse. Alternatively, he should arouse you to the point of fever pitch via manual or oral stimulation before intercourse begins. At that point, any movement in the genital area should put you over the edge, especially if you have a strong PC muscle and flex like mad. Really, isn't this easy? Why make it hard?

The Basic Six Positions

There are six basic intercourse positions and, of course, numerous variations to each of them. They are:

- Woman on top (or female superior)

- Man on top (or missionary)

- Side by side

- Rear entry

- Sitting

- Standing

Female Superior Position (aka Cowgirl)

Considered by sex therapists and women who respond to reader surveys to be the intercourse position most conducive to female orgasm, the woman-on-top position is also a favorite of men. (They like to watch.) She can easily reach her clitoris *and* she controls the depth, angle, and speed of thrusting. In the most common variation of the position, she squats or sits astride (in a riding position) the man, who is lying on his back.

She may lean forward, putting her weight on her hands on either side of his shoulders, or she may lean on one hand, or maintain an upright position, keeping both hands free. Or she may lean backward, if that gives her better G-spot stimulation. A common variation on the position is the "reverse cowgirl," where she faces his feet, not his head.

Missionary Position

In surveys, women usually rate this position more favorably than men do, probably because it allows for hard thrusting. And, yes, women like that! In the most common variation of the position, she lies on her back with her legs slightly parted and he lies on top of her, supporting himself at least partially with his hands.

New Man on Top

This position offers maximum sensation for her with minimal movement for him, and it can help sustain intercourse longer.

She lies on her stomach, legs straight out and spread only slightly. He lies over her, supporting his weight on his elbows. He positions his legs on either side of her. As he enters her, she closes her legs and crosses them at the ankles. Crossing your ankles and holding your legs together enables you to feel the entire length of his penis inside you. As he is thrusting, he's in a great position to kiss your neck and nibble your ears. And you can reach under and play with your clitoris. It's new, it's fun, and it works!

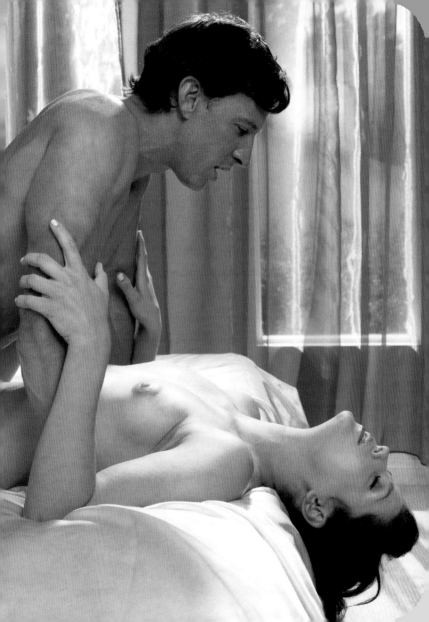

Side-by-Side Position

Often a favorite position for the weary couple—or the semi-erect man—side by side is sometimes called "spooning" and even "stuffing and spooning."

In the basic version of the position, he faces her back. Her buttocks are angled against him as he puts one leg between hers. Or she can lie half on her back, half on her side, drawing up the leg upon which she is lying. He faces her.

For variation, face one another, with legs loosely wrapped around each other. Or keep your legs touching and out straight—with his legs loosely wrapped. In another variation, face one another and she wraps both legs around him, like a lying-down version of stand-up sex.

Rear-Entry Position

A favorite position of the ancient Chinese, rear entry is also a favorite of both sexes in the West today, in spite of its unfortunate nickname, "doggy-style." This position facilitates deep penetration, G-spot stimulation, and hard thrusting and puts her clitoris in a good place for manual stimulation. A nice bonus: Her ass looks its best here, with the little wrinkles and pockets fairly well ironed out. (Who doesn't love that?)

In the basic position, the woman is on all fours with the man kneeling behind her. For variation, he stands behind her and pulls her to the edge of the bed. Standing gives him the ability to thrust even more forcefully—something both partners may want.

In another variation, she lowers her chest to the bed. That changes the angle of penetration. Some women report greater G-spot stimulation in this position.

The Standing Position

Having intercourse while standing satisfies a need we all have sometimes for dramatic, urgent lovemaking. It's a great way to have a quickie or to begin a longer session. You can always slide to the floor and finish in another position.

In the basic version of the position, he squats slightly while she lowers herself onto him. She wraps one leg around his waist and he holds her buttocks. This might be "cheating," but for variation he can lift her onto a kitchen counter, washer or dryer, or any convenient surface when standing becomes uncomfortable.

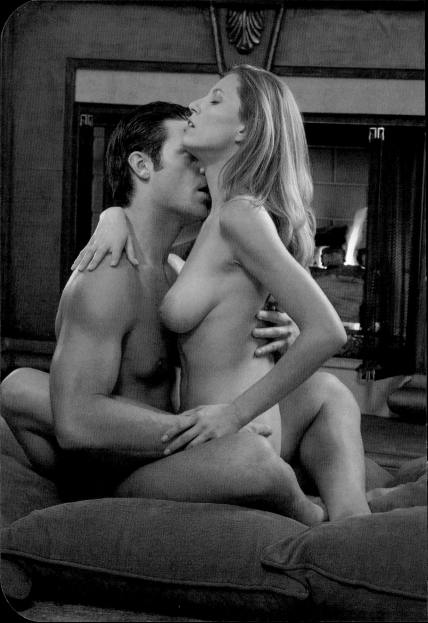

The Sitting Position

There's a lot you can do with this one because it works with different levels of passion. It's good if he's tired or you feel like talking and playing. But it's also good when you just have to sit on him *now*.

In the basic position, he sits in a chair or on the bed with her astride him. Penetration is shallow. Changing the chair also changes the angle and depth of penetration—and her ability to leverage thrusting. A hard-backed kitchen chair, for example, gives her thrusting power, while an overstuffed chair may not.

For variation, she sits on him, facing away from him. Again, that changes the angle and depth of penetration.

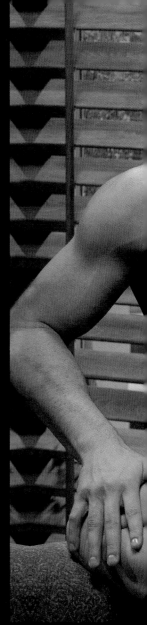

Position
Tic-Tac-Toe

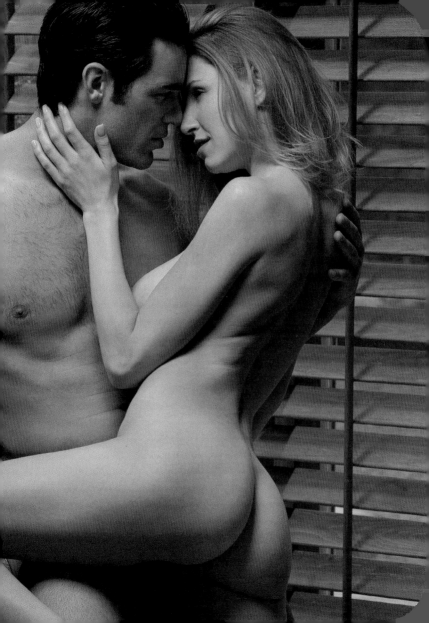

Position Tic-Tac-Toe

The Sexy Setup

Remember playing tic-tac-toe as a child? This naughty version of the same game can be played over and over—orgasms guaranteed! Write your lover a note and tell him you've got a game to play that will test his ability to have multiple orgasms in multiple positions, and there's a bonus prize to boot.

Rules & Tools

You'll need a simple tic-tac-toe game, which you can purchase beforehand or even just draw on a piece of paper. Make a grid using four lines to create nine different boxes. Set a sexy scene and allow for plenty of time for sex play. Alternatively, use the tic-tac-toe game over a span of days, then reward the winner on the weekend!

Playing the Game

Sweet and safe: Try out each of the six basic positions with the goal of having an orgasm in each position. If he orgasms, he gets to mark an **X** in one of the tic-tac-toe boxes. If you also orgasm you get to mark an **0** in one of the boxes. Continue testing the positions and marking the boxes until someone wins the game of tic-tac-toe, then determine a bonus prize for the winner, such as a prolonged back massage, dinner in bed (with both of you naked!), or his choice of the next game to play.

Hot and spicy: Play tic-tac-toe, but use the grid to mark an **X** or **0** each time your lover tries a new technique, is willing to experiment with a new move, or plays with a new sex toy. Play for the winner of three out of five or four out of seven games, then reward the winner with his or her choice of role-play games.

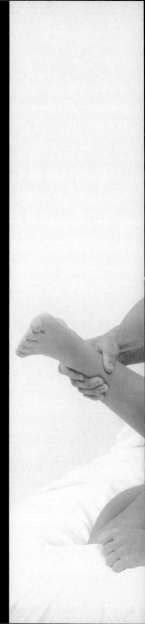

Bag of Tricks

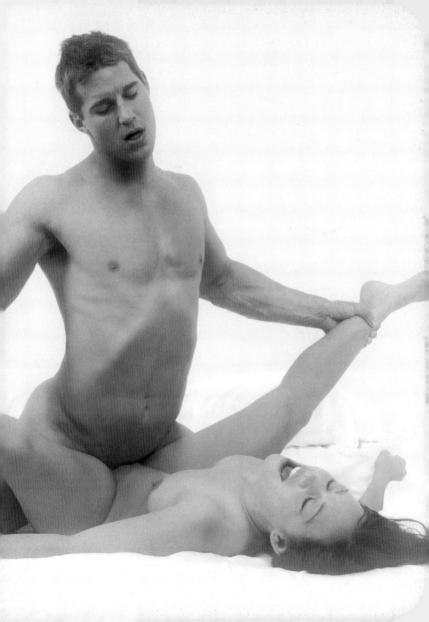

Bag of Tricks

The Sexy Setup

You know that most women don't come via sexual intercourse alone, so tell your lover you've got a bag of tricks you'd like to open up to guarantee you come every time you make love!

Rules & Tools

Bring along your favorite assorted tools for stimulating your clitoris, whether that's your hand, a finger vibe, or his penis. Set a sexy scene, such as a soft rug in front of the fireplace, a pleasure den on your living room floor, or a nest of blankets in your bed.

Playing the Game

Sweet and safe: Kiss, fondle, and caress your lover as you know best, then get naked together using slow and sensual movements. Once you're ready for intercourse, have him enter you manually, then try this simple move for stimulating your clitoris when the space between you is tight. Insert two fingers of one hand between your bodies and form an upside-down V shape with your fingers straddling your clitoris.

Press the V in time with his thrusting. Alternatively, if he's entered you spoon-style from behind, take his fingers and place them in the V shape on the sides of your clitoris. Grind against his fingers as he thrusts from behind.

Hot and spicy: Ready to try some other moves? Kneel together on the bed and have him enter you from behind. Place one hand on the bed frame and use the other hand to masturbate while he thrusts from behind. Have him lie flat on his back, then lower yourself onto him. Once you're in position, lean backward, resting on one hand. Use the other hand to stimulate your clitoris using a finger vibe. Lie on your side, with him on his side between your legs. Wrap your legs around his back. As you control the thrusting movement, have him insert a well-lubed finger between you so he can tickle your clitoris.

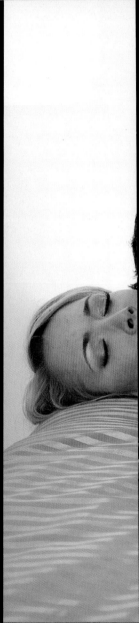

GAME 43

The Bucking
Cowgirl Meets the
Missionary Man

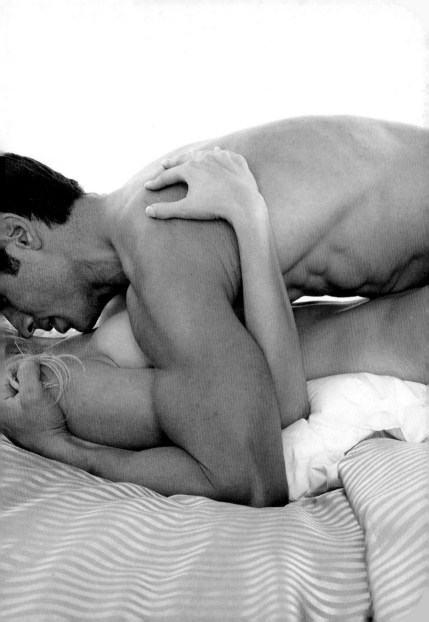

The Bucking Cowgirl Meets the Missionary Man

The Sexy Setup

You know the female and male superior positions by heart: cowgirl and missionary man. Tell your lover you've got a game that's sure to increase the odds of reaching orgasm in either position!

Rules & Tools

Set a sexy scene, such as a soft rug in front of the fireplace, a pleasure den on your living room floor, or a nest of blankets in your bed, and bring along your favorite sex toys if desired. Then let your imagination take over!

Playing the Game

Sweet and safe: Here's how to make the cowgirl an even better orgasm position: Alternate deep thrusting with using the head of his penis to stimulate your clitoris. Move from side to side rather than up and down. When orgasm is imminent, flatten yourself out on top of him, clench your thighs together, and grind your clitoris into him as you flex your PC muscle. In the reverse cowgirl (you facing away from him), ask him to raise one leg and place his foot on the bed. Angle your body so that you are riding his penis at the same time you're grinding your clitoris against his raised thigh. Ready to step it up?

Move in an oval track rather than a straightforward up-and-down riding motion. Imagine you are circumscribing an oval with your body, with the downstroke at one end of the oval and the upstroke at the other. Lean slightly forward as you push down on his penis, stimulating your clitoris. Pull up and move slightly backward on the upstroke, stimulating your G-spot. Use your hand if you need to and don't forget to flex your PC muscle.

(continued on page 336)

Hot and spicy: Make the missionary position even better with this set of tricks: Place a pillow(s) beneath the small of your back to change the angle of penetration to one of greater depth. Lie on your back with your legs up as straight and high as they will comfortably go. He kneels in front of you. This tightens your vagina, providing greater friction for both of you, and it leaves your hands free to play with your clitoris. Lie on your back and put your legs over his shoulders. Lift one leg up and put it over his shoulder or around his back. Put your feet on his chest or shoulders and bend your knees inward, again to change the angle of penetration and control the thrust. Wrap your legs around his waist or his neck for the same reasons. Have him pull you to the edge of the bed and hold your legs as he enters you from a standing position.

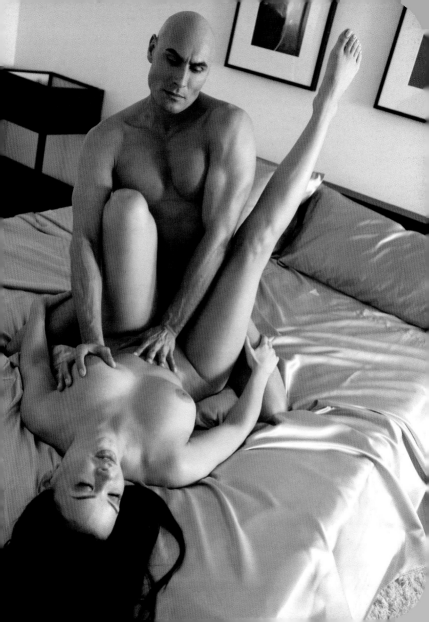

Spoonful of Loving Meets the Backdoor Man

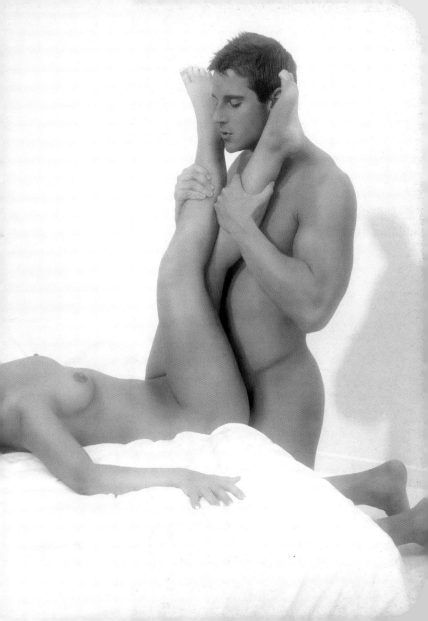

Spoonful of Loving Meets the Backdoor Man

The Sexy Setup

You know the spooning and backdoor positions by heart. Tell your lover you've got a game that's sure to increase the odds of reaching orgasm in either position!

Rules & Tools

Set a sexy scene, such as a pleasure den of soft blankets, furs, and pillows on your living room floor. Dim the lights or light some candles and bring along your favorite sex toys if desired.

Playing the Game

Sweet and safe: Here's how to make side by side, also known as spooning, a better orgasm position: Either you or he should stimulate your clitoris. Start by adding a vibrator—this is a great position for vibe play because your hands are free. Make this your go-to position when he's tired, but you want sex. Masturbate first until you are highly aroused, then let him enter you from behind. Touch yourself while he thrusts away, and try to time your orgasm to his!

Hot and spicy: Ready to freshen up that old doggie-style position? Try these moves for better orgasms: Lower your upper body so that your chest touches the bed. This elongates your vaginal barrel, making a tighter fit for his penis. If he typically grabs your hips or ass and controls the thrusting, ask him to caress your vulva and finger your clitoris while otherwise remaining relatively still. Then you thrust back against *him*. Alternatively, try the rear-entry position lying down, with you on your stomach. Clench your thighs together after he enters you and lift one leg for deeper penetration.

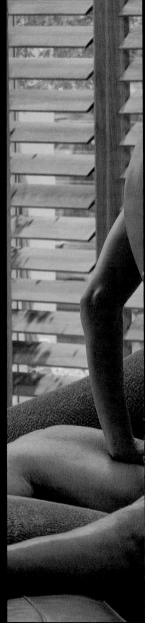

Sitting Lotus Meets the Stand-up Man

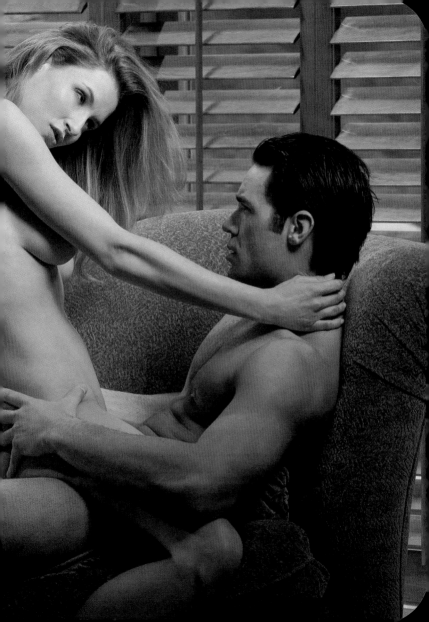

Sitting Lotus Meets the Stand-up Man

The Sexy Setup

You know the sitting and standing positions by heart. Tell your lover you've got a game that's sure to increase the odds of reaching orgasm in either position!

Rules & Tools

Establish an erotic mood with candles, wine, sexy clothing, or music—whatever turns you on and gets you tingly all over. Bring along your favorite sex toys or silk ties for gentle bondage if desired.

Playing the Game

Sweet and safe: Here's how to make the sitting position even hotter: Have your lover grasp your buttocks firmly, then lean backward as he thrusts. Add a vibrator, especially a vibrating cock ring on him or a strap-on vibe for you.

Hot and spicy: Use these moves to bring your standing position to new heights of passion! Change the depth and angle of penetration by doing it on the stairs, with you one step above him. Alternatively, stand in front of him, facing in the opposite direction, and bend slightly forward. You'll feel more G-spot stimulation this way. Last but not least, sit on the kitchen counter, washer or dryer, or a high bar stool—whatever is the right height for him to enter you.

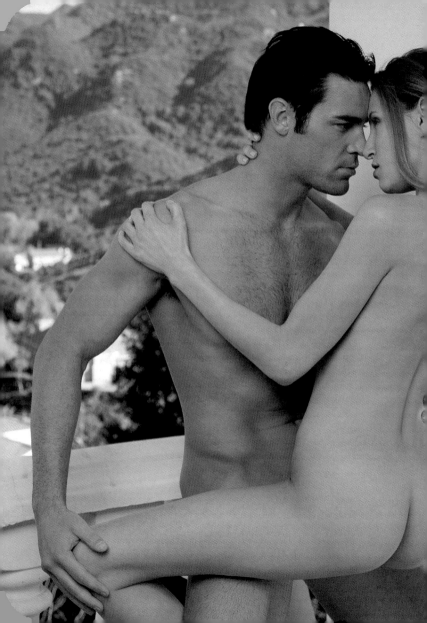

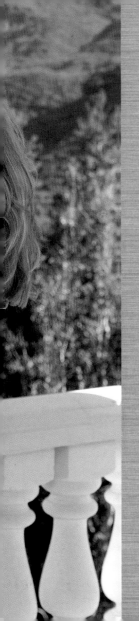

CHAPTER 10

Come Together: The Orgasm Connection

Reaching orgasm at the same time during lovemaking is a wonderful thing. Postorgasmic chemicals racing through your bodies enable you to gaze into your lover's eyes with renewed affection and appreciation. Coming together can make the orgasm connection more intense, but don't berate yourself if it doesn't happen.

Achieving Simultaneous Orgasm

The keys to simultaneous orgasm are communication and timing, and couples in long-term relationships are more familiar with each other's bodies and sexual responses than strangers are. You shouldn't feel pressured to make this happen, but trying to bring your orgasms together can be fun even if the timing doesn't work out. Try each of the following three techniques to see which one works for you.

Stretch Out Foreplay

If you are very aroused by the foreplay (either manual, oral, or a combination) *and* are comfortable in giving yourself—or asking him to give you—continued manual clitoral stimulation during intercourse, you can have an intercourse orgasm fairly easily. With a little planning, you can have simultaneous orgasms. To make it happen, do the following.

Extend the warm-up. Hold off on intercourse until you are both at the "high fever" state of arousal. You know the signs: panting, sweating, flushed skin, that look in the eyes. Don't move to intercourse until you get those signals. Then move together in a state of close communication, with your eyes open and your hands on

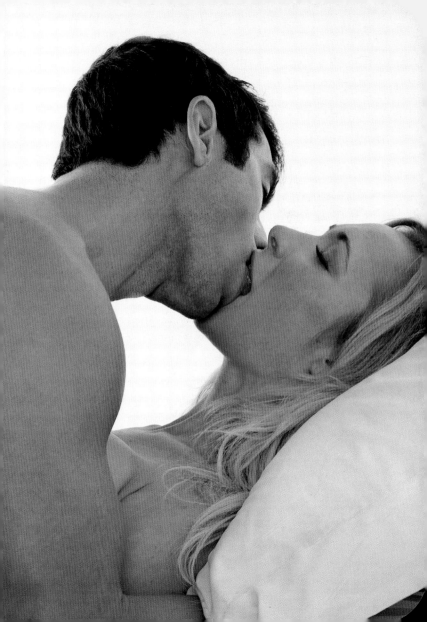

each other's back, buttocks, or thighs ready to indicate "faster" or "slower." If one of you is closer to orgasm than the other, that person stops moving and signals through a sexy code phrase like "too hot" or a touch, such as gently placing your hands on the other's hips and pushing your bodies slightly away from one another. Still connected though not moving, the partner on the verge kisses, caresses, and strokes the other. Look into one another's eyes now if you are comfortable doing that, because eye contact during intercourse will let you gauge how close your partner is to release, helping you time the movements. The more dilated those pupils are—and that glazed and unfocused look—the closer you are to orgasm. Now move together again to bring about simultaneous orgasms. (And you can see why couples who know one another well can make this work.)

Why does it work? The partner who signals for a brief halt in stimulation gets the slowing down he or she needs while continuing to give the erotic attention the other needs to keep his or her arousal building. The less aroused partner continues to receive the kissing, stroking, and caressing he or she needs to catch up. This method of letting the "faster" partner focus attention on the "slower" partner until they are in sync again dramatically increases the odds that they will reach orgasm at the same time.

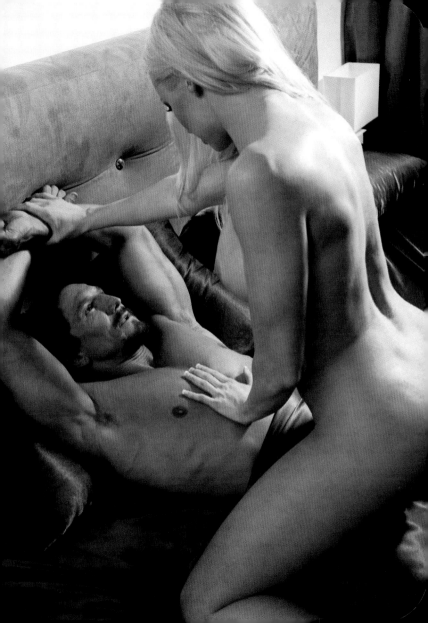

Forget "Ladies First"

To have a simultaneous orgasm, she should forego the prerogative of the "ladies first" orgasm through cunnilingus. Here's how to make it happen.

When he has stimulated you either orally or manually to near orgasm, pull back from the attention he is lavishing on your body by gently taking his face in your hands and pulling your hips back at the same time. As soon as you send him this physical signal, he'll understand that you are ready for intercourse. He, on the other hand, may need a little extra stimulation to catch up. Ask him if he wants oral or manual pleasuring, and give him enough to bring him up to your speed. Get into the "69" position. That will give you enough additional stimulation to sustain your high while you're bringing him along. *Now* you're both ready!

Use eye contact to gauge each other's arousal. Also use the physical cues to control the timing—for example, grasping one another's hips to encourage faster or slower movement as needed.

This method works because, when you start intercourse at a high level of arousal, you're where he typically is at the beginning. He doesn't have to hold back.

The Adapted C.A.T. Position

The Coital Alignment Technique (C.A.T.), an adaptation of the missionary position that puts his full weight on her, has been touted as the no-fail simultaneous orgasm position. The problem? It's very uncomfortable for a woman if her partner is bigger than she is. Here's how it's done.

She lies on her back and he enters her. With his pelvis higher than hers, he lies on top of her, putting his full weight on her body. (If he's a lot taller, his chin will be resting on top of her head because he has to move his pelvis as high as it will go while sustaining the intercourse connection.) She wraps her legs around his thighs, resting her ankles on his calves. They move their *pelvises only* in a steady rhythm without speeding up or slowing down until they reach orgasm together.

You can adapt this basic position, taking some of the weight off her and allowing face-to-face contact, no matter your heights. While keeping your pelvises locked and her legs around his thighs as described above, he supports most of his weight on his arms. Another way to open up the C.A.T. and lift his weight off of her is for him to grasp the headboard, using that to support his weight and leverage his movements against her. Or you can reverse the C.A.T., with her on top, lying flat against him, pelvises locked, his legs wrapped around her body. In any variation, speed up or slow down that "steady rhythm" to suit your own timing needs.

This method works because your clitoris is stimulated directly and you can reach orgasm during intercourse alone. Plus the constraints the position places on his movement naturally slow him down, which makes you more likely to be in sync. He moves less vigorously and at the same time gives you that steady stimulation right on target.

Achieving Sacred Sex

Sacred sex, also known as sexual ecstasy or "high sex" in some Tantric circles, is a way of making love that is supposed to incorporate body and soul in one ultimate erotic experience. Seminars and workshops on the techniques of sacred sex have proliferated in the past decade. You can book hotel getaway weekends that include afternoon classes. Bookstores devote entire sections to Tantra, the five thousand-year-old Eastern belief system that united the searches for ecstasy and enlightenment in ancient India. Here's an overview of the basics of sacred sex.

The Tantric Twist

The Tantrics worshiped the god Shiva and his consort, the goddess Shakti, who they believed united the spiritual and the sexual. Their traditions included a variety of techniques then unknown in Western culture.

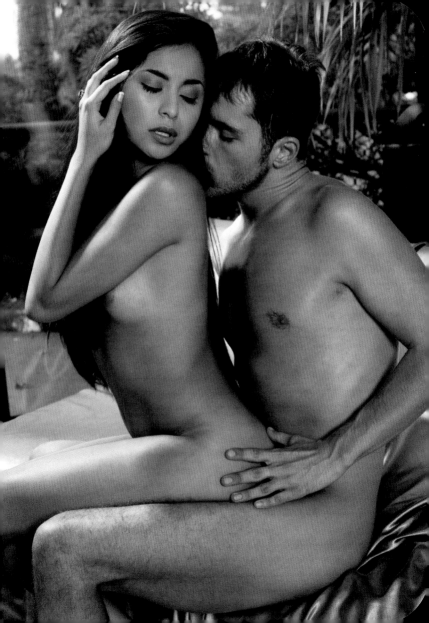

Those traditions influenced people in other societies, including in Tibet, China, and the Arab world. Eventually, they made their way West but didn't really make an impact on American society until the second half of the twentieth century.

The American way of lovemaking is goal-oriented and straightforward: Get to intercourse, orgasm, and good night. The Eastern way is about prolonging pleasure, extending orgasms, and expanding the orgasmic experience until the body seems suffused with orgasm. It's the quickie versus the long, slow love-in.

Most of us won't immerse ourselves in Tantra. (If you want to read further, the world authority on Tantra is Margot Anand, and I recommend her books because they are accessible, well-written, and interesting.) We can, however, adapt some of the techniques and use them to enrich our sex lives.

Techniques for Slowing Him Down and Speeding Her Up

Tantra may be so appealing to Western lovers because it tackles the two common mind-sets that come together to create unsatisfying sex: As a boy, he learned how to masturbate quickly to avoid getting caught, while she absorbed the lesson that, for her, an orgasm wasn't nearly as important as the "feelings of closeness" generated by lovemaking. That is the basis for the kind of sex that led to the quip, "Yes, the prince will come—too soon!"

By contrast, on the Tantric path to ecstasy, lovers are supposed to experience:

- Prolonged love play

- Prolonged intercourse

- More intense orgasms

- Longer, or extended, orgasms

- Suffused, or whole body, orgasms

- Intense emotional or spiritual connection

The techniques for making these expanded, extended, and whole body orgasms are best learned during masturbation. Expanding orgasm takes it beyond the places in the genitals where you usually experience it. Sometimes the techniques are referred to as "stretching" his orgasm and "spreading" her orgasm. If you master these techniques, they simply make your orgasm feel a little more diffuse, bathing the genitals and immediately beyond in pleasure. And they feel stronger!

Expanding His and Her Orgasms

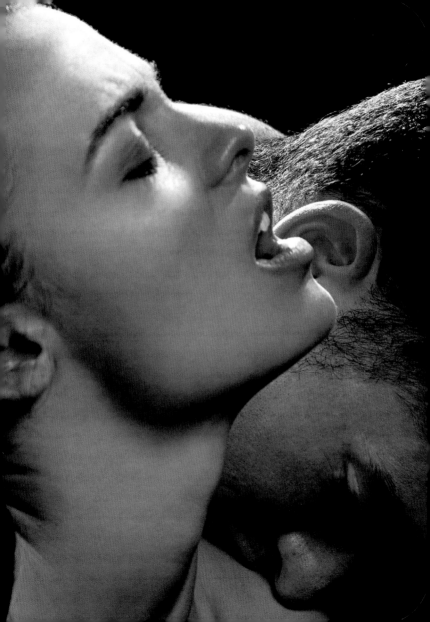

Expanding His and Her Orgasms

The Sexy Setup

If you love the idea of orgasm, then chances are you'll relish the idea of expanding an orgasm so it becomes a full-body or even body-mind-spirit experience. Write your lover a romantic note and tell him you've got a game that will *spread* your orgasm beyond the usual boundaries and *stretch* his orgasm into new territories!

Rules & Tools

You can use these masturbation techniques alone beforehand for practice, but they can also be used with your lover for communicating how you want to be touched. Set a sexy scene for your love play, such as a nest of blankets in your bed or a soft rug set in front of a roaring fire. Bring along extra pillows for good positioning and viewing and your favorite sex toys if desired.

Playing the Game

Sweet and Safe (for her): Using your fingers or a vibrator, masturbate in a comfortable position. As soon as you become highly aroused, use one hand to massage the area of your vulva, inner thighs, and groin with light, shallow strokes. Imagine that you are spreading your arousal throughout those areas. Continue the massage throughout your orgasm, imagining you are spreading your orgasm into your body. After orgasm, continue rhythmic stroking of your genital area. Feel the orgasm continuing to spread throughout your body for several seconds after it normally would have dissipated.

Sweet and safe (for him): Have your lover masturbate without ejaculating as long as he can. Ten to fifteen minutes is a reasonable goal, though this may not be possible not the first time. Have him do this by stopping or changing strokes when ejaculation is imminent. Have him count the contractions he feels upon ejaculation, normally between three and eight. Note the level and order of intensity. Typically the strongest contractions will be at the beginning. The next time he masturbates, again delay ejaculation as long as possible. This time when he comes, have him flex his PC muscle as if he's trying to stop ejaculation. Then have him continue stimulating his penis very slowly—or do it for him—while squeezing throughout the ejaculation, thus pushing the sensations on and on.

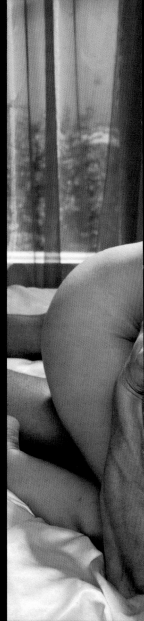

GAME 47

Expanding
Orgasms
Together

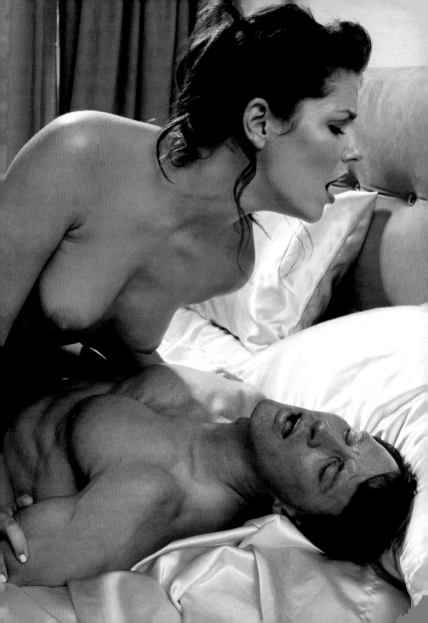

Expanding Orgasms Together

The Sexy Setup

If you've mastered the technique of expanding your orgasm through masturbation, you're ready to step it up and expand your orgasms together. Text your lover and tell him you've got a game that's sure to redefine simultaneous orgasm!

Rules & Tools

Take a cool, not hot, shower together. Your skin should be cool to each other's touch as you begin.

Playing the Game

Sweet and safe: Lie on the bed side by side, facing one another, with your legs entwined in a scissors position. Insert his flaccid penis into your vagina. Remain still. If necessary, put your hand around the base of his penis to keep it inside until he has a moderate erection. (But don't work to make him have one!) Breathing deeply, try to remain motionless for fifteen minutes. During this time, caress each other's faces, necks, and upper bodies, and make frequent, prolonged eye contact. Whisper terms of endearment. Are you feeling a sense of erotic peace? Now begin moving together. He should be thrusting slowly and gently and you should match his pace with your pelvis and hips. Kiss deeply. As you move your bodies, use your hands to stroke each other, working upward from one another's genitals. Imagine that you are spreading fire with your hands. Resist the desire to move faster when you reach that agonizing point of being "almost there." You want to stay on the verge for as long as possible—until you realize that you are having an orgasm that seems to last forever.

Hot and spicy: Repeat the sweet and safe game, but try to remain motionless for thrity minutes. As you begin moving together, make your thrusting motions as slow and prolonged as possible. Kiss deeply with your eyes open, and try to maintain eye contact as you begin caressing and stroking each other. Whisper how your hands are spreading fire from his penis upward, or as his hands glide from your genitals to your buttocks, nipples, belly, and back again. Hold on to the slow, drawn-out pace as long as possible—your goal is to reach the edge and stay there as long as possible before you both achieve orgasm. Try to maintain eye contact the entire time for the ultimate intimate connection.

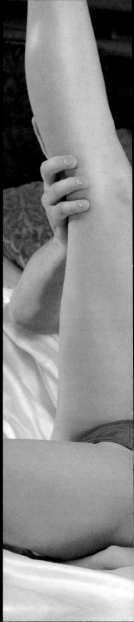

GAME 48

Karezza

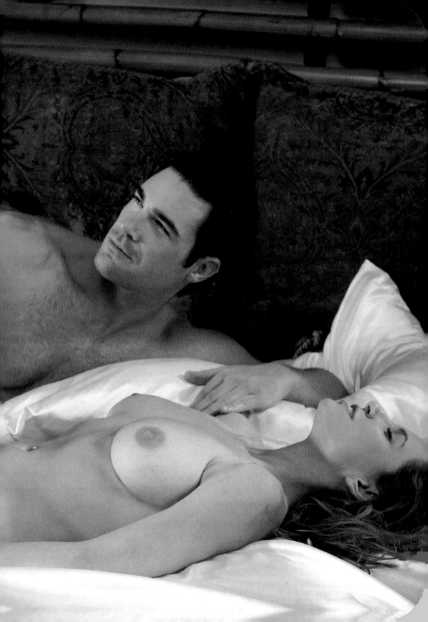

Karezza

The Sexy Setup

An Italian word that means "caress," Karezza was developed by an American physician in 1883. As a technique for prolonging intercourse, Karezza is simple and effective and can be practiced in any position. It also encourages extended orgasm—and what woman doesn't like the promise of that reward?

Rules & Tools

Any intercourse position can work for Karezza, but man on top or missionary is least likely to work, so woman on top or side by side are better choices.

Playing the Game

Sweet and safe: The key is to dramatically limit your genital movement. You do not move inside your lover unless you become flaccid. Then you take only shallow strokes to revive your erection. Your lover is allowed to move, including thrusting her hips against yours and contracting her PC muscle around your penis. No matter how excited she gets, you should only take sufficient thrusting strokes to maintain an erection. Using the masturbation technique of expanding or "spreading," she can encourage the spread of her orgasm throughout her body.

Hot and spicy: Hold the lovemaking embrace until she has had several orgasms, then move with more energy and satisfy yourself!

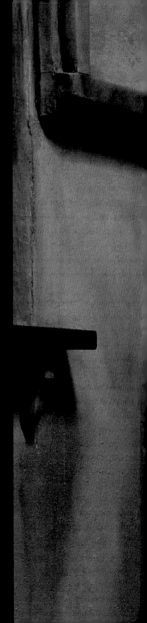

Kabbazah

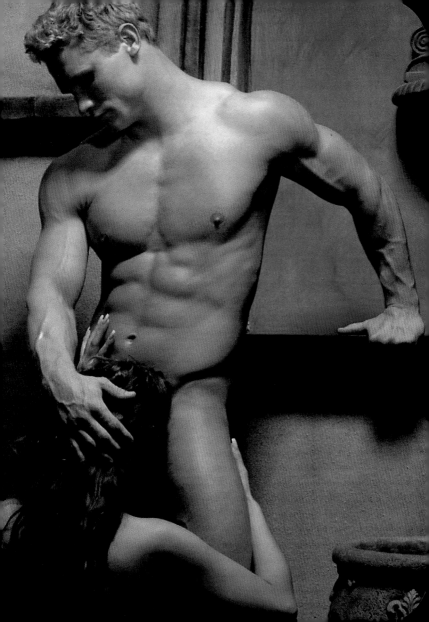

Kabbazah

The Sexy Setup

Kabbazah was developed thousands of years ago in the Middle East. A woman who had mastered the French art of *pompoir* (control of the PC muscle) was called a *kabbazah*, or "one who holds." Kabbazahs were the best prostitutes in many Eastern countries, including China, Japan, and India. This game won't be a hard sell to your lover: Just tell him you've learned an ancient trick practiced by prostitutes that's guaranteed to intensify his pleasure!

Rules & Tools

There are two absolute requirements for Kabbazah: He must be in a relaxed and receptive state of mind and body. His passivity is crucial. This is not the kind of sex you have when you are desperately tearing each other's clothing off. Second, you must have a virtuoso vagina. Don't even try this until you have diligently practiced Kegels for a period of three weeks to a month.

Playing the Game

Sweet and safe: Begin in the female superior or sitting intercourse position. You should stimulate your lover until he is just erect, not highly aroused. Then insert his penis, but instruct him not to move his pelvis *at all*. You should also strive for no pelvic movement, confining all movements—or as much as possible—to your PC muscle. You may, however, caress and kiss each other. Flex your PC muscle in varying patterns until you feel his penis throbbing, which should occur approximately fifteen minutes into Kabbazah. At that point, he should be highly aroused—so let him take over and orgasm.

Hot and spicy: Play the sweet and safe version of the game, but when you feel his penis throbbing don't hand over the controls. Instead, time your contractions to the throbbing of his penis, clenching and releasing in time with him. In another ten to fifteen minutes, he may experience a longer, more intense orgasm than ever before.

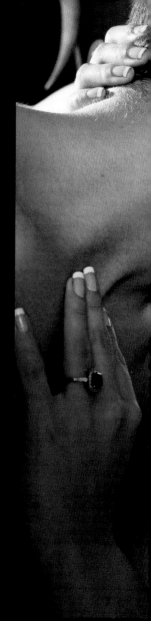

The Whole Body Orgasm

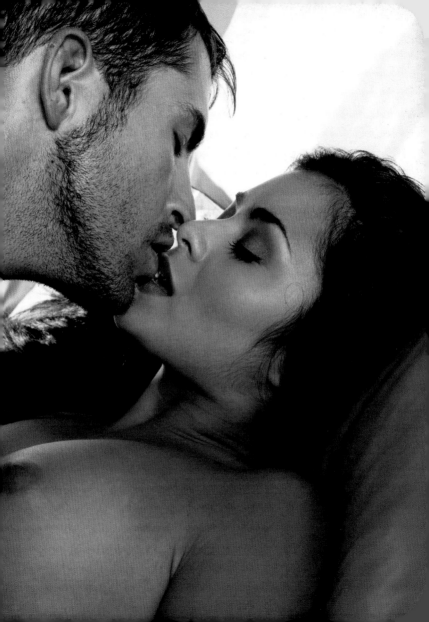

The Whole Body Orgasm

The Sexy Setup

The whole body orgasm is the result of intense connections on three levels: emotional, sensual, and sexual. Tell your lover that in order to reach this state you'll need to jourey through three doors together.

Rules & Tools

The kiss is particularly intimate and sacred in Tantra, and the belief is that during the kiss, the soul and energy of one partner flows into the other, and vice versa. To experience a whole body orgasm you'll need to master the Tantric yoga kiss the Yabyum.

Playing the Game

Sweet and safe: To master the Tantric yoga kiss, do the following. During intercourse (in any position), have him practice one of the methods described earlier to delay his orgasm and ejaculation. When you feel your own orgasm is imminent, signal him to stop moving. Then sit in the middle of the bed with his penis inside you, legs wrapped around each other, moving as little as possible. Pressing your foreheads together, breathe into each other's mouths. As he exhales, you inhale, and vice versa. Prolong this "kiss" until remaining still is no longer an option. Movement will trigger orgasm. The long, slow arousal period and the emotional intensity of the kiss can combine to make your orgasm feel like a whole body experience.

Hot and spicy: The Yabyum, a Tantric version of the Western sitting position, is a must-try for experiencing whole body orgasm. It is highly touted by sexologists as the ultimate position for prolonging male arousal and intensifying lovers' intimate connection. Sit in the center of the bed facing each other. Wrap your legs around one another so you are sitting on his thighs. Place your right hands at the back of each other's neck, your left hands on each other's tailbones. Now stroke each other's back, using upward strokes only. Look deeply into one another's eyes as you kiss with eyes open. Put his semi-erect penis inside your vagina so it exerts as much indirect pressure as possible on your clitoris and makes G-spot contact. (You can sit on pillows rather than his thighs, if necessary, to get the angle of penetration right.) Perform the Tantric kiss described earlier. Rock slowly together while continuing to rub each other's back and sustaining deep eye contact. Maintain this position until you both orgasm.

Alternatively, try the Passion Flower: As in the Yabyum, start in the center of the bed, facing one another. Wrap your legs comfortably around his body. You can either sit on his thighs or on pillows positioned in front of him. Splay your legs out straight or bend them at the knees, whichever is more comfortable for him. Place your right hands on each other's neck and your left hands at the base of each other's spine. Stroke each other's back, using upward strokes only. Look into each other's eyes and kiss with eyes open. Continue kissing and stroking until you're both highly aroused. Insert his erect penis into your vagina so that the shaft exerts as much indirect pressure on your clitoris as possible. Rock together, slowly rubbing each other's backs and kissing deeply. You may reach orgasm quickly in this position. After your first orgasm (or sooner, if you don't feel orgasm is imminent) try this variation: Have him sit on the bed with his legs open wide. You should lie back on the bed, facing him, with your body between his legs. He lifts your ankles up against his shoulders and enters you at a comfortable angle. Keep your thighs closed, creating a tighter grip on his penis and use one hand to stimulate your clitoris.

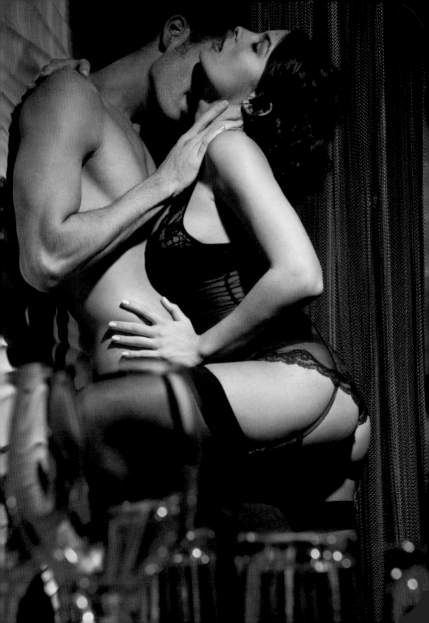

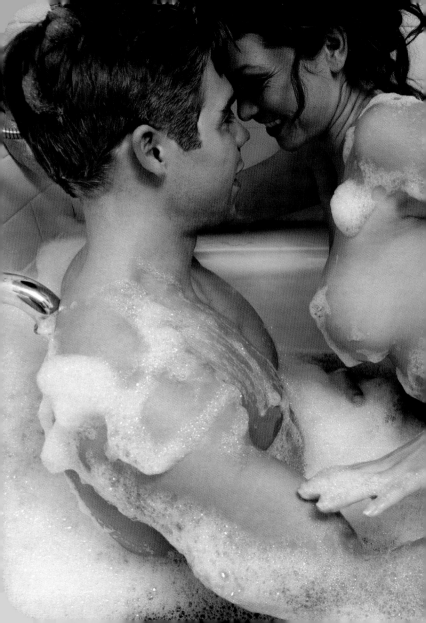

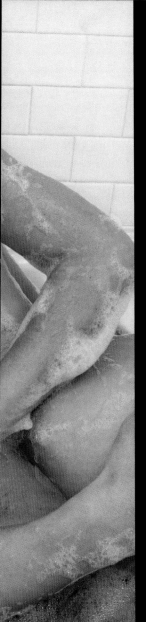

Your
Game
Checklist

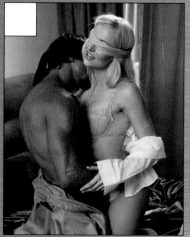

1 Tap into Two Senses

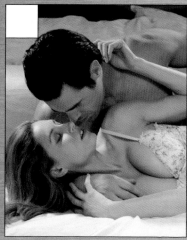

2 Anatomy Test

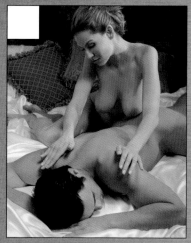

3 Crisscross Applesauce

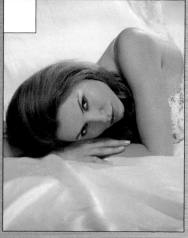

4 The Art of Seduction

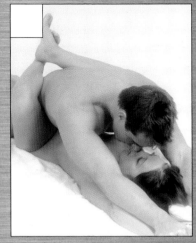

5 Touch Me Here

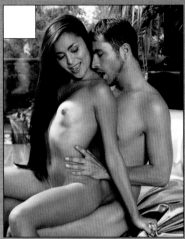

6 Flex Test

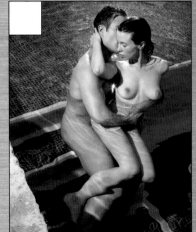

7 Bring Out the Big Cats

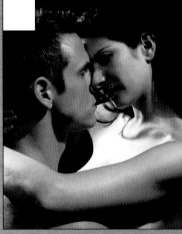

8 Playing with Kundalini Fire

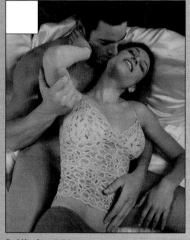

9 Kissing 101

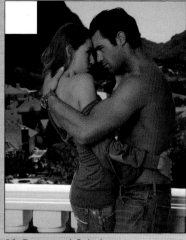

10 Bump and Grind

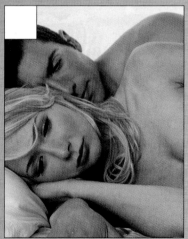

11 Think Yourself Off

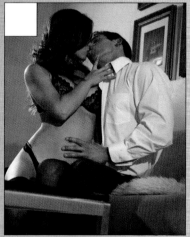

12 Couple Fantasy Encounters

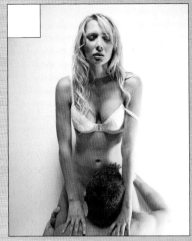

13 The Queen of Orgasm

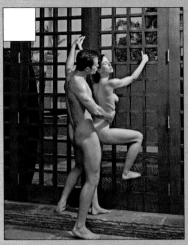

14 Handyman Cum Calling

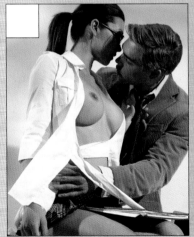

15 Back to School

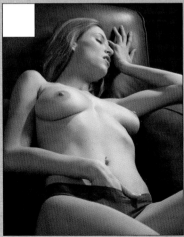

16 Mutual Masturbation

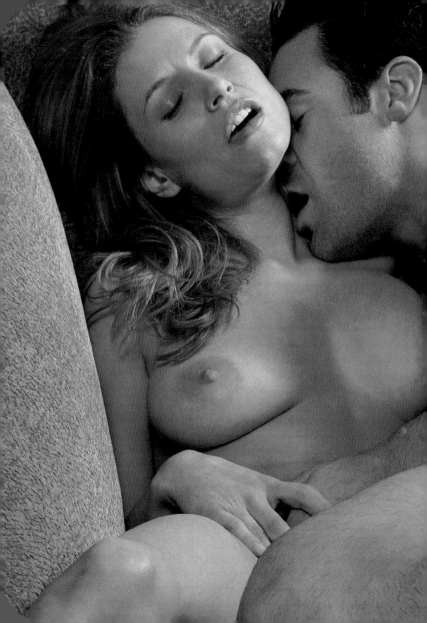

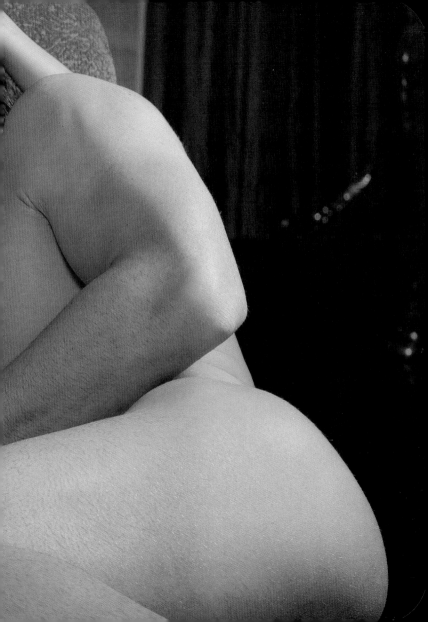

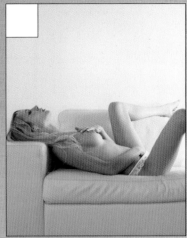

17 Masturbation Slave

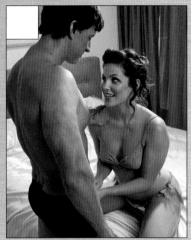

18 Learn His Strokes

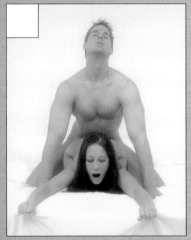

19 Door-to-Door Vibrator Salesman

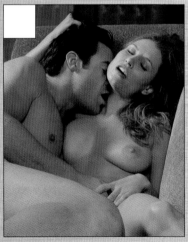

20 Finger Fun

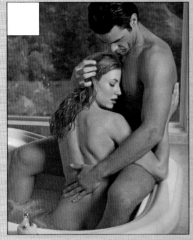

21 Queen of Foreplay

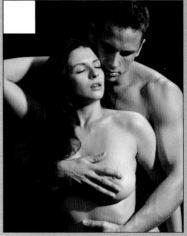

22 King of Foreplay

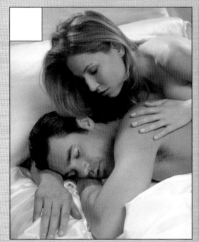

23 Reviving a Fallen Soldier

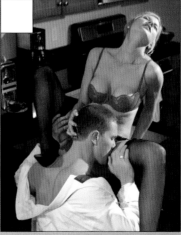

24 Preheat the Oven

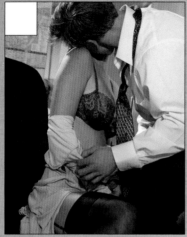

25 Variations on a Theme

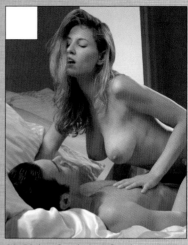

26 Pick a Card, Any Card

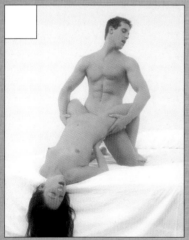

27 Connect the Dots

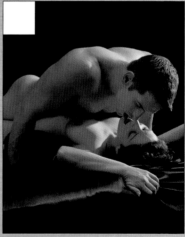

28 Hot Spot Intercourse

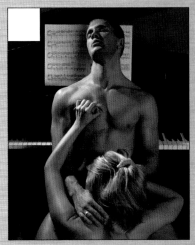

29 Drawwwww Out His Pleasure

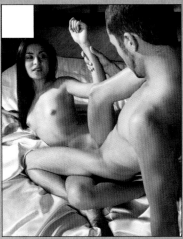

30 Spike My Oh!

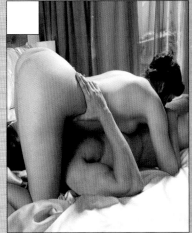

31 Classic 69 (and Then Some!)

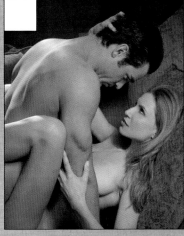

32 Queen for a Day

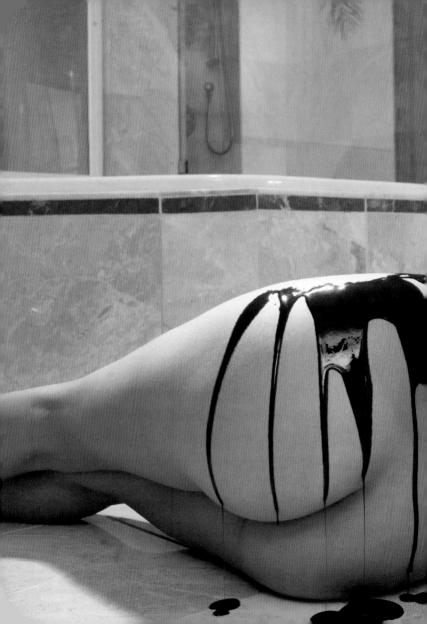

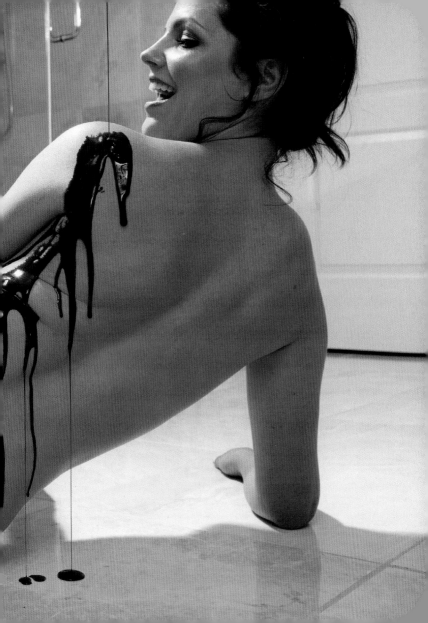

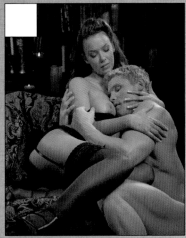

33 Oral Sex Slave

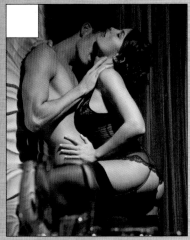

34 8 Days a Week

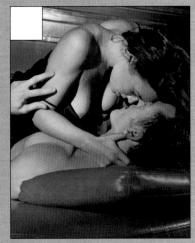

35 Stranger Danger

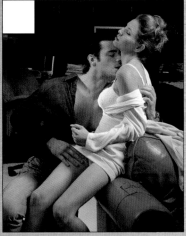

36 Dress for Quickie Success

394 • The Little Book of the Big Orgasm

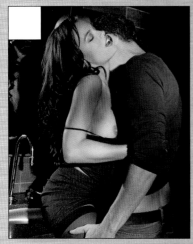

37 Quickie Chinese Menu

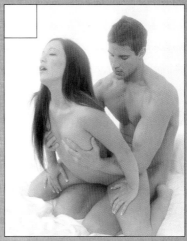

38 Anal Play 101

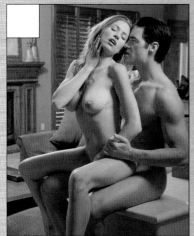

39 Beyond Doggie-Style

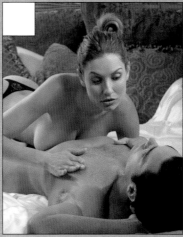

40 Backdoor Woman

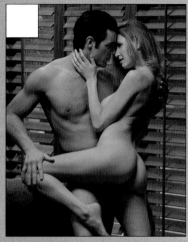

41 Position Tic-Tac-Toe

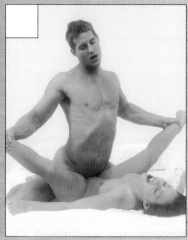

42 Bag of Tricks

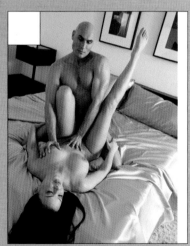

43 The Bucking Cowgirl Meets the Missionary Man

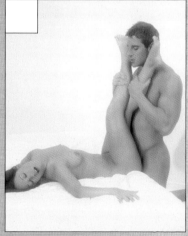

44 Spoonful of Loving Meets the Backdoor Man

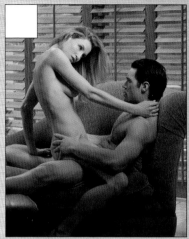

45 Sitting Lotus Meets the Stand-Up Man

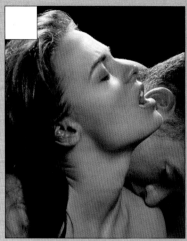

46 Expanding His and Her Orgasms

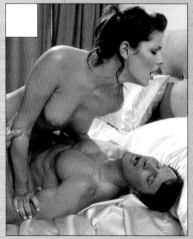

47 Expanding Orgasms Together

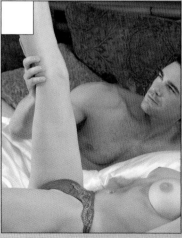

48 Karezza

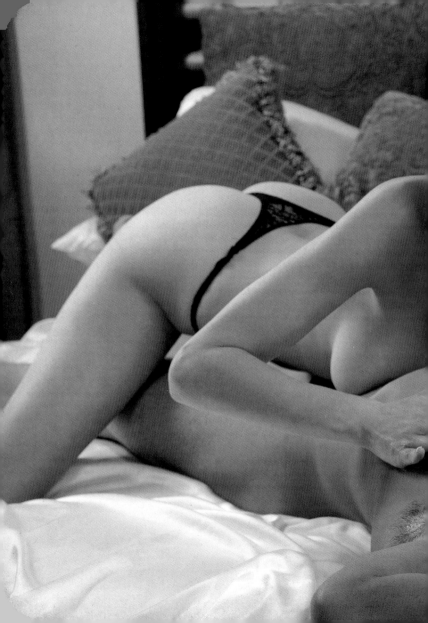

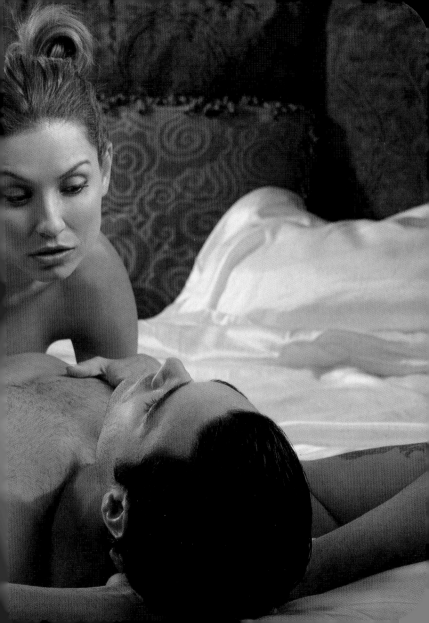

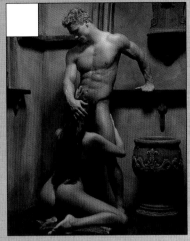

49 Kabbazah

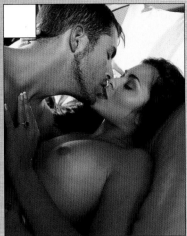

50 The Whole Body Orgasm

About the Author

Susan Crain Bakos is an internationally recognized sex authority and author of eighteen books, including *The Sex Bible: The Complete Guide to Sexual Love* and *The Orgasm Bible*. She has been writing about sex for more than two decades, with her work appearing in such magazines as *Redbook, Cosmopolitan, Men's Health,* and *Penthouse*.

A former contributing editor and columnist at *Penthouse Forum*, Susan has worked with such legends as Dr. Ruth Westheimer and Helen Gurley Brown and has interviewed thousands of men and women about their sex lives. She has also appeared on *Oprah*, Good *Morning America*, and numerous other television and radio shows. She lives in New York City and holds steadfast to the belief that every woman should own a veritable wardrobe of vibrators and have at least one orgasm a day.

Visit her blog
www.sexyprime.typepad.com

INDEX

G